Conscious Eating

or

HOW TO STOP EATING
IN RESPONSE TO EVERYTHING!

Conscious Eating

or

HOW TO STOP EATING
IN RESPONSE TO EVERYTHING!

*Sharing their struggles and triumphs together, five women
join a* DIETLESS™ *group and discover their emotional
connections to weight loss.*

What happens next surprises them all!

by
Carol Asada, Ph.D. & Joanna Haase, Ph.D.
Founders of DIETLESS™

Manufactured in Canada
Cover Design by Beth Farrell
Interior by Krishna Gopa
Photographs by Jeff VerHoef

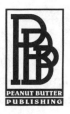

Published by Peanut Butter Publishing
Pier 55, 1101 Alaskan Way, Suite 301
Seattle, WA 98101-2982
206-748-0345 • e-mail: pnutpub@aol.com
http://www.pbpublishing.com
Denver, Colorado • Scottsdale, Arizona
Portland, Oregon • Vancouver, BC

LCCCN: 97-066409
ISBN: 0-89716-752-X

CONTENTS

Acknowledgments . . . . *page* VII

About the Authors VIII

Introduction X

1 The Journey Begins 1

2 Week One: Weight Loss Without Dieting?
    Conscious vs Unconscious Eating 13

3 Week Four: Emily vs Three Dozen Cookies
    Feeling Deprived Leads to Weight Gain 37

4 Week Eight: What Do You Mean I Have a Choice?
    Customizing Food to Lose Weight 63

5 Week Ten: What's Missing in My Life?
    Identifying the Other Hungers 91

6 Week Thirteen: I'd Rather Be Fat Than Exercise!!
    Responding More Accurately to Other Hungers 121

7 Week Fifteen: Where's My Money?
    The Connection Between Money & Weight 151

8 Week Seventeen: I Have a Food for Every Feeling?
    Recognizing the Relationship Between Food & Anger 175

9 Week Eighteen: But Wait a Minute, I'm Not Done Yet !
    The End and The Decision 201

∽ DISCLAIMER ∾

THIS BOOK IS A WORK OF FICTION, designed to illustrate similarities among women who struggle with weight and food issues. It is based upon the authors' knowledge gained from their professional training, education, research, and experiences. The characters portrayed herein are not actual case studies. Rather, the characters were created as a means of illustrating and discussing the themes common to women with weight and food issues. They are not intended to represent specific persons or to suggest that the events described actually occurred. Any similarities between the characters and their stories in this book and any real person is purely coincidental.

ACKNOWLEDGMENTS

THERE ARE NOT ENOUGH WORDS to express our deepest gratitude and profound thanks to Eldonna Lay for all her time, energy, and talents she gave so generously to this project. She helped us turn an idea into a reality.

For reading our manuscript, we are most grateful to Gay Serway, Merideth Hattrup, and Virginia Levinson. Their interest and suggestions were invaluable to us.

We greatly appreciate all the support and encouragement we received from our editor, Anne Melley. She was a delight to work with.

Many thanks to Elliott Wolf for his professional guidance through the publishing maze. He made an overwhelming process more organized and manageable.

Our deepest appreciation go to Margie Martin and Bonnie Asada, who were constant sources of ideas, suggestions, and loving support. From the bottom of our hearts we thank you!

We are forever grateful to Christopher Thomas for his creativity and generosity to all our endeavors.

And last but not least, we wish to thank our husbands John and Jim for what can only be described as everything!

✑ ABOUT THE AUTHORS ✑

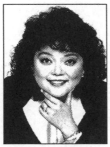

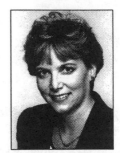

Carol Asada   Joanna Haase

D R. CAROL ASADA is a licensed clinical psychologist with a private practice in the San Diego Area. Since 1981, her areas of expertise have included Binge Eating Disorder, Bulimia Nervosa, and Anorexia Nervosa.

Dr. Joanna Haase is a licensed Marriage, Family and Child Therapist with a private practice in the Los Angeles area since 1985. Her areas of expertise include Bulimia Nervosa, Anorexia Nervosa, and Binge Eating Disorder.

*We dedicate this book to all the women who have participated
in our program from its earliest inception to the present.
They are an inspiration to all women looking for their
emotional connection to weight loss.
We applaud their courage and their progress.*

∽ INTRODUCTION ∾

MORE THAN 35 BILLION DOLLARS are spent annually on diet programs and diet products, yet more women are overweight today than ever before and the numbers are rising. These statistics reflect the real problem facing so many of us who want to lose weight. Diets and diet products only serve to hook us into a vicious cycle of deprivation, weight loss, and subsequent weight gain. After years of being caught up in this cycle, we end up feeling like failures in our attempts to maintain weight loss.

This book was written to proclaim to ourselves and the world that we are not failures! Traditional weight loss methods have failed us in that they never guide us to discover our emotional connections to weight loss. The answers are not found in calories, fat grams, or diet pills.

We believe that permanent weight loss cannot be achieved without trust in our bodies, conscious eating, and a safe, supportive environment. As babies we knew when we were hungry and we knew when to stop because we were full. But somewhere along the way, we stopped listening to our bodies. We began to eat for our heads, ignoring whatever our bodies truly needed. Eventually all communication broke down and we ate when and what our minds told us to. Once we begin to trust that our bodies will tell us what it needs, we can re-learn the physical cues for hunger and satiety. When we know what physical hunger feels like, we can identify all the other hungers we try to satisfy with food.

The awareness of physical hungers and other hungers is important because it lets us see all those times we eat when we aren't physically hungry. We call this unconscious eating, and unconscious eating leads to weight gain. Conscious eating is eating only for physical hunger which results in weight loss and weight loss maintenance.

Once we are conscious of other hungers and have defined more accurate ways of taking care of them, then we have the choice to do it or not. Each time we choose to take care of those other hungers more accurately, we decrease the amount of unconscious eating and the extra weight begins to come off.

Another important aspect of weight loss maintenance is to create a safe, supportive environment that will support change. Careful attention to these aspects of our lifestyle will bring to awareness other areas of deprivation and blocks that keep us from achieving our goal of permanent weight loss.

When we decided to write this book, we chose to present our DIETLESS program in novel form rather than the usual "How To" format. We wanted you, our readers, to see and experience the process of approaching weight loss from a psychological perspective – working on behaviors, thoughts, feelings, and physical awareness all at the same time. We felt that this goal would be impossible to accomplish with intellectual exercises. As you read about the journeys of these five fictional women, we hope you will be able to identify with their life stories and become more aware of all the possibilities, choices, and answers that lie within each one of you.

CA & JH

CHAPTER ONE

The Journey Begins

FIERY REDHEAD in a dark green pantsuit made her way through the hotel lobby. Halted momentarily by a bank of closed elevator doors, Kate Dvorak jabbed impatiently at the "up" button. When that didn't bring the desired result, she stepped back and used the next few minutes to rearrange the wildly patterned scarf around her neck. Seconds later, a sizeable group of men and women were assembling around her, as impatient as she. When a door finally slid back, everyone moved forward as if pulled by strings. Inside, Kate quickly turned around, which set the dangling combination of rolled wire and brightly lacquered metal on her ears ajingle. The sound pleased her; reminding her again that they turned out to be every bit as pretty as they'd appeared on the shopping channel! To keep her spirits up, she shook her head to set them off again. Unusual earrings and scarves were great for pulling people's attention away from her bulky body. From her experiences with other weight reduction gurus, however, she doubted that the fashion ploy would fool anyone upstairs. And then the elevator stopped.

With the parting of the doors, Kate and several other women stepped out to find three women standing beside a registration table in the hall directly ahead. This had to be it, Kate told herself. Suddenly, the joyful tinkle of her earrings didn't matter.

Reaching the table behind the other women who had also exited the elevator, Kate read the name tags of the three greeters. Two were the program founders she'd heard on the radio the other day. What they'd said about diets not working was the reason she was here, even though it was Saturday, an especially busy workday in the construction business. The other person's name tag read "Marti Lenox, Ph.D., Clinical Psychologist." Each of them was, Kate thought, an attractive woman; one appearing to be in her mid-thirties, the other two in their forties. It was a relief, she thought, to see that they weren't the usual buffed-out, skinny weight-loss promoters. Hoping against hope that this program would help her finally get rid of her excess weight, she felt like this was her last chance. Her marriage was on the line. So, although past failures made Kate want to turn around and put as much geographical space between herself and them as possible, Kate pasted a smile on her face and bravely stepped forward to accept a packet of information.

Past the welcoming committee and in the meeting room, Kate saw rows of upholstered armchairs. Choosing one in the last row, she sank down and sighed. She then became aware of being comfortable, a highly unusual feeling to experience in most meeting rooms. Looking down, she saw how roomy the chair was. Making sure no one was watching, Kate wriggled around a bit, enjoying a sense of unexpected freedom. But then what had happened earlier crowded out that pleasure. So she sighed again as her mind returned to what she'd been thinking about all morning—Ed.

As was becoming alarmingly usual, Ed had been too hung over to get out of bed this morning, so it was up to her to go into the office to get the day started. She worried about what kind of example Ed was giving to everyone, but was grateful that no one seemed to notice. The rest of the staff was already at the office and working when she arrived. Up until a few years ago, Ed had felt the same way about the business. Now, he was becoming more and more irresponsible, and not only at work, either. For the millionth time, Kate wished Jody was still around. For fifteen years they'd lived next door to each other, raising their kids together and sharing nearly everything: graduations, weddings, holidays. They'd been there for each other through all of it, the ups and the downs. After their parenting days were over, they'd had a ball traveling together and exploring the far corners of the country. Kate really missed being able to run next door, to share a homemade pie, or to just get away from it all for a few hours. But that had all stopped nine years ago. Jody and Don had just moved away without warning or explanation. Memories of that fateful day were still fresh in Kate's mind: seeing the moving truck outside their house, the quick goodbyes, the promises to keep in touch, and then standing alone in front of her house as they drove off. They were gone and out of her life in what felt like a split second. Kate had wondered then if she'd ever recover from the shock.

Kate made it through the first few months without Jody on sheer willpower. She'd even taken pride that she hadn't once given any outward indications that she was hurting... nor that she was becoming increasingly anxious about Ed's odd behavior. Six months later, she'd started crying – for no reason at all. Even today, just remembering how miserable she'd felt made her feel bad all over again. But, back then, she had actually cried, and for so long and hard that she couldn't even get out of bed. Fortunately, at the time, Ed was running both the construction jobs and the office, but it took its toll. He'd gotten downright mean on a couple of occasions, and once he even told her that he was tired of her "fat-ass lying around." Kate had forgiven him for that, of course. But the truth was that when her housebound days turned into months, it became clear even to her that something was seriously wrong. So, even though she hated going to doctors, she went in for a check-up. Beyond giving her a bad time about carrying so much extra weight, the doctor found nothing physically wrong with her. Suspecting depression, he referred her to a psychiatrist. Thank God Ed never found that out – he surely would have had something snide to say, and it was bad enough without having to endure that, too! Sitting there in that beautiful hotel room, Kate closed her eyes against remembering her one and only psychiatric session. It hadn't worked.

Had she recently suffered a loss? That's what the psychiatrist had asked her. But, even as her brain was framing a denial, Kate found herself sobbing, "My best friend!" It was as if it had happened only yesterday instead of months before. She wept, "Jody moved away a year ago. It happened so fast that we didn't have a chance to talk. And I haven't heard a word from her since." She continued, "Jody and I did so much together. She was the only person in the world that I've ever felt close to."

"What about your husband?" the psychiatrist queried. Startled into subduing her tears, Kate had replied, "Well, I don't feel comfortable telling him much of anything, anymore."

That had brought on a whole series of questions about Ed and their relationship. How she hated to admit that Ed wasn't interested in anything she did outside of the office. When the psychiatrist suggested that it must be difficult to communicate with someone like that, the understatement nearly made Kate snort out that she and Ed hadn't "communicated" in a long time. Pressed to give some sort of answer, Kate explained that they'd been married right out of high school, Ed had quickly risen from a journeyman carpenter to become owner of a small but successful construction firm. "I run the office, and he gets the contracts and then oversees the jobs," Kate said. "He's really good at what he does." Then she went on to explain that about a year and a half ago, he'd won a huge contract. Business had been growing ever since. Sensing that this success might be a source of another loss, the psychiatrist kept inquiring about the relationship. Kate remembered feeling uneasy talking about her husband, but she couldn't understand why he'd been acting so differently around her. So she tried covering it all up by reasoning that it was all her fault. "Over the last few months, I haven't been a good wife," she said. "And I've gained a lot of weight. So he's had good reason to be mad at me."

The psychiatrist asked, "So when did Ed begin to change?" The question started Kate thinking. Surprisingly, she remembered that it hadn't happened after their friends moved away. Rather, he had begun acting strangely right after winning that enormous contract. It was like nothing would please him, like she never did anything right. His sharp tongue didn't stop at home, either. "One time, in front of all our employees, he called me something that he knew would hurt me" Her voice dropping, she whispered, "He called me worthless."

"Why does that word bother you?" asked the psychiatrist. Kate's reply was spoken in such low tones that the doctor had to lean forward to hear it. "It's what my father called me all of my life," Kate had whispered. Even now, years later, Kate felt the old sadness well up.

She never went back to the psychiatrist. What good had it done? That was one of the things bothering her about today: the program had been developed by psychotherapists. What did all that psychobabble have to do with losing weight? Brought back to the present, Kate opened her eyes. Surprised to find the room half full, she wondered how all these women had arrived without her being aware of it.

Emily Hardesty had been one of the arrivals. Only 9:30 in the morning and I'm already exhausted, she was thinking as she dropped into the chair right in front of Kate's. Of course, Emily reminded herself, she'd been working hard since 4:30 getting ready for the birthday celebration, marinating meat and putting final touches on her husband's favorite cake. Like all of her parties, this one had to be perfect because this is the pressure she always placed on herself. Both sides of the family would be there, which meant twenty-three adults and children. Cooking for that many was a lot of work, but it was also fun because they enjoyed it so much. Well, everyone but her parents, who always seemed so upset about the amount of food she prepared. No one else thought it was too much and, besides, setting an abundant table was something Emily had vowed she would do since childhood. She was nine when she decided that when she was grown up, no one would ever leave her table hungry. And no one had. But because of her weight, she herself never ate a single bite. Her food was carefully limited to diet fare. But, if what the two doctors had said on the radio program were true, she might not have to do that anymore. What they had talked about was a no-diet approach to permanent weight loss. No forbidden foods. No rigid exercise regimens. Instead, a careful look at the real reasons people eat when they aren't hungry. And they had also mentioned that women use food to feed other hungers in their lives. These were new thoughts, and Emily sat thinking about them.

Fifteen miles away, Margaret Hemming was buttoning the top of her best Diane Freis look-alike dress. She looked just long enough in the mirror to make sure that its floating panels were hanging right. Another quick glance allowed her to check her hair. Happy with the way it looked, she started to smile. Then she remembered why she was so dressed up on a Saturday morning, and her half-smile disappeared. Was this going to be one more exercise in futility? Yet, if she didn't attend this preview, she might as well forget ever getting her figure back. Sighing, she left a note on the kitchen table for her son, Donnie, picked up her purse, and went out the door. But when her Lexus reached the end of her driveway it was obvious that she wasn't going anywhere. Lined up, bumper to bumper, was a long line of cars, vans, and trucks filled with children in sports uniforms. Spring sports season had arrived. From all over town, kids and their parents were descending upon ballfields and school playgrounds, and their dedication was going to make her late. Margaret hated being late more than anything. Maybe, she thought, this was a sign. Maybe she wasn't supposed to go.

Back in the conference room Emily was deep in thought. Those thoughts were distracted when she heard her stomach growl. Embarrassed, she took a quick look to see if anyone else had heard it. Relieved that no one was paying attention, her thoughts returned to those other hungers the psychologists had talked about. The only hunger Emily knew was physical hunger because she always felt that starvation was right around the corner – which was crazy for someone who weighed as much as she did. So, she was the tiniest bit intrigued by the suggestion that she might be feeding some nonphysical hungers. Was that possible? Emily wondered. Whatever. She was ready to consider anything that would prevent her from constantly thinking about food. Even now, she was sorry she hadn't brought some rice cakes in from the car. To take her mind off them, Emily forced herself to take another look around the room. When her eyes reached the doorway, they stopped. A woman with the most beautiful dress was standing there, and Emily found herself wishing she had something like that in her closet.

Had Margaret been aware of this admiration, she would have felt even more self-conscious than she did. Distressed at being late, she'd hurried herself into walking so fast that she was perspiring. Worse, her feet were swelling inside of her shoes and she could just feel the blisters forming. It was terribly uncomfortable. Suspecting that she looked as bad as she felt, Margaret found herself worrying. Would everyone think that she looked this bad all the time? What made that so galling was that it was far from true: always, she was so impeccable, precisely as Bob and his associates had come to expect.

Being supportive of her husband had been the center of Margaret's life since she and Bob decided to marry nearly thirty-three years before. Bob was a senior when he proposed to her in her sophomore year of college. She dropped out of school at the end of that term and got a job so they could get married. Upon his graduation, Bob went on to law school and she kept working, even after Craig was born. Bob was approached by a couple of law firms even before he'd graduated. He decided to go with the group he considered the most prestigious because they were the best in corporate law. This job allowed Margaret to quit work just in time for the birth of their second son, Donnie. Shortly after that, they purchased their first house. It was small, but definitely a place they could call home. She furnished it with the turn-of-the-century arts and crafts style Bob liked. Her choice would have been French provincial, but she had wanted to please her husband.

That had pretty much been how she'd handled everything, from the types of cars they bought, to the organizations she joined, to the kinds of foods she cooked. Now, with the boys grown and Bob still traveling, she had more freedom to do what she wanted. But that only left her feeling empty. She didn't know what to do with all that spare time. And she didn't think that joining another organization would be the answer, either.

Still not sure that she'd made the right decision in coming, Margaret made her way into the meeting room and sat down. After a few minutes, she realized how dry her mouth felt. She had noticed a refreshment table at the back of the room, but didn't want to make a further spectacle of herself by getting up and getting a drink. So she opened her purse and searched out a mint. Doing that gave her the first pleasure she'd felt all morning, for tucked into the side pocket of her purse she found Devon's pre-school photograph. How lucky she was to have such a beautiful grandchild. And luckier still, with the divorce and all, to have Cheryl allow Devon to visit several days a month. Of course, next fall when Devon went to kindergarten, that would change. But Margaret didn't like to think about that. So she thought about the grandparents she knew who'd lost touch with their grandchildren when their children separated.

Margaret had been careful not to take sides in the divorce. In fact, she had even admitted to Cheryl that Donnie still had a lot of growing up to do. However, she also pointed out that the divorce had been very difficult for him – which was true. Just from the way he acted, Margaret knew it was hard for him to move back into his old bedroom after living in an apartment of his own. But, with his debts, he had no other choice. Then, to make matters worse, he had to buy a new car because Cheryl got their car in the settlement. When Bob found out that Margaret gave Donnie money for the down-payment and had co-signed the loan, he was furious. But Margaret didn't know what else she could have done. Sighing, she turned her attention to the materials in her lap. Quickly, she became so involved that she didn't notice the strawberry blonde who slipped into a seat a few chairs away.

Julie Martin's rush through the lobby equaled Margaret's. Unlike the older woman, however, she was unaccustomed to the elegance of hotels with chandeliers and marble floors. Her first reaction was to question whether she should have come. Next came the fear that she wasn't wearing the right kind of clothes. Ordinarily, that wasn't a consideration – kids paid little attention to what librarians wore. But adults judged you differently. Still, she was desperate enough over her weight that she couldn't turn back. So she hurried to the three women at the table and whispered, "I'm Julie." Then, taking the materials they offered, she walked quickly to a chair and sat down.

Sneaking peeks around the room, Julie saw tree ferns in the corners, subtly painted wainscoting on the lower third of the walls, rows of framed botanical prints above, and solidly built chairs covered in cheerful floral prints. The setting reminded her of an encounter she'd read about the night before – of lost love recovered in a darkened room just like this. She smiled, recalling that unlikely romance. Who would have thought that the daughter of a wealthy merchant would be swept off her feet by a pirate. Of course, he wasn't a common buccaneer – his manners were far too sophisticated. Oh, Julie sighed, her reading was such a wonderful escape from the people she had to deal with at the library. And, at home, it gave her something to do after the kids were in bed and Tom was on the computer. She smiled again, reviewing the fictional rendevous. Then, for no reason at all, she was reminded of what she'd heard on the car radio just a few minutes ago. A commercial promoting candy and cards for Mother's Day.

Her mother preferred cigarettes to candy, and the messages inside most cards about gratitude, kindness, and understanding didn't describe Julie's feelings at all. What was she supposed to be grateful for – love, support, acknowledgment, validation? Julie received none of that. Ever! However, she found herself always trying to find ways to win her mother's love. Dreading the upcoming weekend as she did, Julie wondered if things would have ended up this badly if Dad had stayed.

After the divorce, life was never the same. Julie and her brother, Eric, had to deal with not only the loss of their father but also the loss of the feeling of being part of a family. Their mother moved everyone to Grandmother's house. Because Mom was rarely home, it was as if Julie and Eric had lost their mother, too. Grandmother had let them know from the moment they arrived how they were inconveniencing her. So, living in her house never felt like living in a real home. Julie found refuge in her books, and Eric took off with his friends. By his second year in junior high, he was either drunk or drugged out most of the time. Now 34, Eric couldn't keep a job and Mom couldn't admit that he had a problem. But Julie knew that her mother was mainly concerned with maintaining the figure of a 20-year-old so she could continue to be attractive to men. All of this was so embarrassing that Julie never mentioned having either a mother or a brother to anyone outside of her immediate family. It was her own private terror that if people found out about them, they might think badly of her, too. But there was no time to worry about that now. The program was starting.

For the next hour, the roomful of women heard data that startled them, conclusions that reinforced what they'd suspected, and statistics that provided hope. Perhaps the most encouraging piece of information was that gaining back lost weight didn't mean that they were failures – it simply proved that diets don't work! One poor lady supported their statements by saying, "Every time I gained the weight back, it just proved that something was wrong with me. But I'm glad to hear that it wasn't my fault; now I understand why the weight came back." One of the founders then said that if they used the information they received today, the women would be taking their first step towards accepting their own power to change what they didn't like about their struggle with weight. A latecomer standing beside one of the chairs in the last row frowned. It was an intriguing idea, but what did it mean? Then, glancing down, she realized that she hadn't removed her hospital name tag reading "Bobbie Boone, M.D., County Hospital Emergency Room."

CHAPTER TWO

Weight Loss Without Dieting?

Week One: Conscious vs Unconscious Eating

S AN EMERGENCY ROOM PHYSICIAN, Bobbie often worked as many as 60 hours a week. For that reason, her days off were usually spent sleeping. But today was the first Wednesday of the month, so she was headed for the country club to have lunch with her mother. Steering her aged van through traffic, the physician thought back a few weeks to the Preview. Some of what the psychologists said had really struck home. She wished she could talk about those things with her mother, but Camilla would say, "For heaven's sake, Bobbie, you're the doctor – don't you already know how to lose weight?"

Well, maybe she should, Bobbie thought. But she didn't! What she did know, she learned in medical school. And med schools were run by men who, knowing little about either women or their weight issues, continued to hand out the same old advice: eat less and exercise more. Well, she was living proof that the old formula didn't work. But then, neither did anything else! All of which reinforced what Bobbie had come to believe twenty years before: that her weight resulted from a lack of character. Whenever she did lose weight and the lost pounds ricocheted back the instant she stopped dieting, it reaffirmed her belief. Why that happened she hadn't known until the Preview when the therapists said "Rebounds in weight were to be expected after a long period of deprivation!" Two weeks later, Bobbie was still marveling at how it all worked.

It's all a simple matter of survival. Because the body doesn't know the difference between diets and famine, its reaction to each are the same. When the body doesn't get enough calories it assumes there is a famine and begins a process of adjusting the metabolism, storing needed calories for later, and prioritizing what gets the nutrients first. Going through countless cycles of dieting and not dieting, the body never has a chance to adjust to the fact that food is plentiful. So it continues as if there is a famine by slowing its metabolism and storing nutrients in the form of fat, thereby making it harder and harder to lose weight. But then, when the two psychologists said that women sometimes use food to deal with feelings, Bobbie almost closed her mind to everything else they said. She heard other attendees say that they had suspected all along that there was more to their weight than too many calories and too little exercise. Still, Bobbie didn't get it – maybe because she'd never investigated that side of herself. Was it possible? Did her feelings have something to do with all this weight?

Lost in her thoughts, Bobbie saw a large green expanse of lawn ahead. The entrance to the country club. Looking down at what she was wearing, she sighed. She had worn the only clothes still fresh from the last dry cleaning delivery. They were clean and didn't smell of the hospital. Even at that, Camilla Boone would find something wrong with her outfit – she always did!

Back when she turned fourteen, Bobbie came to realize how her metamorphosis from a skinny kid to a chunky teenager embarrassed her mother. For a woman dedicated to keeping her own figure, having an overweight daughter was humiliating. How, Camilla brooded, do you explain something like this to your friends?

Well, you couldn't. So when lectures didn't work, Camilla, determined to turn her daughter into a social butterfly, put her on a stringent diet. And it worked – for a while. Then Bobbie started gaining weight again. Camilla responded by going back to square one. First she restricted Bobbie's food, then put her on another diet. When that didn't work, Camilla resorted to bribery.

Whenever Bobbie lost a few pounds, Camilla showed her delight by taking her shopping in nearby Chicago. But Bobbie didn't like the clothes her mother chose, and she didn't like where she was supposed to wear them. Bobbie hated going to the club's monthly cotillions her mother thought so important. Not that the kids were openly rude or mean, but they hurt her feelings just the same. So, Bobbie went to the parties. As she watched everyone else laugh and kid around, she waited for what she knew was coming.

Before she'd started attending what she termed the "cotillion rigmarole," Bobbie had never had to play the unpleasant little game called "place card tag." She learned fast, although she never got used to the snickering that accompanied her search for a place to sit. She had to go up and down the table in front of everyone because one – or more – of them had moved her place card away from themselves and next to someone else. If that person discovered the trade, they moved the card on to another person. That was because no one wanted to be associated with a fat girl, and Bobbie was all too aware of that. She even understood it. Unfortunately, her mother didn't! So, more and more, Bobbie retreated into her studies. Her teachers, of course, loved her. It was they who encouraged her to take the most demanding classes.

Academic success was Bobbie's salvation. Like her father, she was blessed with a mathematical mind, and she won all the honors in math, chemistry, and biology. And it was in the exciting world of academia that she discovered genetics. What that meant for her, she found, was that she'd inherited the body shape, size, and intellect of her father's family. Hoping that this would help her mother recognize and respect their differences, she mentioned it to Camilla – once. It only made the woman step up her efforts to make Bobbie more socially acceptable. This, of course, doomed Bobbie to blunder her way through the rest of her high school nightmare. Luckily, her sister, who was only three and a half years younger, became a freshman the year Bobbie was a senior. The spitting image of Camilla, Melanie was pretty as well as smart. Not smart enough to intimidate boys or outshine the more popular girls, but smart enough to fit in. With Melanie to showcase, Camilla lessened the pressure on Bobbie. That, however, didn't stop Bobbie from trying to please her. To that end, Bobbie decided to use the best of what she had and made the dean's list all four years in college. She even lost some weight. Then she made another decision that she hoped would make her mother proud. It only upset Camilla more when Bobbie announced with pride, "I've decided to become a doctor." Camilla made no effort to hide her dismay. It wasn't bad enough that Bobbie was still single. Now, she wanted to go on to med school? When, Camilla wondered, was Bobbie going to find a husband and start a family?

Throughout Bobbie's years in medical school, Camilla repeatedly asked her who she was dating, Bobbie tried to explain that she had no time to do anything but study. Working as hard as she was, she continued to lose weight. When Bobbie graduated, she served her internships in New York, and then was hired by the hospital in her hometown. By then, Melanie was suitably married and following in her mother's charitable footsteps.

Having a slimmer Bobbie back in town made Camilla redouble her efforts to push her eldest into more social situations. That's why she started their monthly luncheons. As the club was used by men of all ages and professions, she hoped that Bobbie might finally see someone who interested her. Despite the fact that Garth was now living with Bobbie and that they had been in relationship for a couple of years, Camilla insisted they continue their luncheons. They'd been meeting this way now for three years, years in which Bobbie had been steadily gaining weight.

Arriving a little late, Bobbie bent over to kiss her mother on the cheek and sat down. Right away, Camilla started talking about the decorations they'd chosen for the club's next gala ball. "You'll have to come, Bobbie," she said. "Everyone who's anyone will be there." Nodding, Bobbie beckoned to the waiter and they ordered. Only when their salads arrived did Camilla realize that Bobbie had ordered the steak caesar. "Oh Bobbie," she sighed, "All that meat, cheese, croutons, and dressing! How can you eat all those calories?" Deciding not to respond, Bobbie kept eating. But she hoped that Camilla wouldn't say what she usually said: "No wonder you have a weight problem – don't you have any self-control?" All too well, Bobbie knew what was important to her mother: being born into the right family, traveling with the proper crowd, marrying well, and keeping one's looks. But, fortunately, Camilla said none of that this time. Instead, she paid meticulous attention to thoroughly chewing each dainty bite of her own garden salad. What Bobbie didn't know was that her mother was watching her devour every bite and wondering why her daughter had to eat so much and so fast. If she changed her ways, Camilla thought, maybe dear Garth would marry her. Inspired by that thought, she chose her words carefully, then spoke.

"You know dear," she said, "you and Melanie both have such pretty faces." Widening her eyes as if she'd just remembered, she asked, "Did I tell you about Melanie? She lost five pounds last week just by giving up salad dressings, gravies, sauces, and sweets. And she says it was easier than she ever thought possible!" Bobbie nodded to let her mother know she'd heard, but she was thinking that Camilla would never understand that she and Melanie had inherited completely different genes. Well, she sighed, at least she hadn't told her about the new program. She'd never understand!

Not getting a response from Bobbie, Camilla gave up. Bobbie finished her salad in record time – and in continuing silence. But even as she was swallowing the last bite, Bobbie thought, there she goes again – trying to tell me how to lose weight. Suddenly, Bobbie wondered what was on the dessert tray. She couldn't ask the waiter, of course, because that would really send Camilla over the edge. So Bobbie glanced at her watch, then gasped, "Oh my. I've got to be at the hospital in ten minutes." Kissing her mother again, Bobbie fled.

Pulling out of the club lot, Bobbie could no longer deny an all-consuming need to fill her mouth with something sweet and chocolatey. Something smooth covering a center of caramel and nuts would reward her for having survived the mother-daughter lunch. Knowing that there was a convenience store close to the hospital, Bobbie drove there and parked. Inside, she headed for the candy section from which she selected the biggest candy bar she could find.

Waiting until she was back in the car to begin eating, Bobbie polished it off in the short time it took to drive to the hospital. But as she got out of the car and turned to lock it, she looked inside. There was the wrapper crumpled up on the seat. Suddenly, she felt a sense of self-loathing. Maybe Mother was right, Bobbie thought. She always said I was fat because I didn't have any will-power. Brooding about this all the way across the lot to the emergency room, Bobbie wondered if she'd ever lose the weight. But once inside the door, she remembered it was her day off, so she left with lightning speed before anyone could ask her to stay. By the time she reached her office, she was bone-weary. As she collapsed into her big, leather chair, she realized that the only part of her that was working was her brain. And it was saying that she was hungry again. Sitting there, Bobbie considered her situation. Slowly, she got up and went to her desk. Opening the top drawer, she used both hands to push aside the candy wrappers, memos, a fingernail file, and some reports. Finally she uncovered it: the folder from the Preview.

Reluctantly, Bobbie stared at its bright cover, afraid to open it up. Would anything inside explain her uncontrollable hunger? More to the point, would this program be able to stop it? And, how was she going to justify paying for yet another weight-loss program? On the other hand, she mused, maybe she ought to give it a try. What did she have to lose but a few dozen pounds? And, I promise, she told herself, that if I haven't lost anything by the end of the first month, I'll know that the psychologists' program is no better than any of the others. But this time, she wasn't going to tell her mother, Garth, or anyone else what she was doing. If she failed, no one would know. Except, of course, the other women in the group. And that was another thing bothering her. She'd been in enough fat camps and vacation groups in junior high and high school to last a lifetime. Oh well, she told herself, I'll give it a try. And she picked up the phone.

* * * * * *

In her office a week later, Marti glanced at her watch. She had ten minutes before it would be time to begin the first meeting of the newest group. Using that time, she thought about the weekly consultation meeting she'd had with Carol and Joanna, when they discussed the background of the newest participants in the program.

Marti was ready to see to it that each woman learned to listen to herself as closely as she listened to others. By doing that, the women would begin to recognize similarities in their perceptions, experiences, and attitudes. It was through the sharing process that each of them would begin to pull out long-forgotten parts of themselves. But what all that required, Marti knew, was that everyone feel comfortable speaking honestly and listening to others with open hearts. Empathy and diplomacy helped that process along. Marti thought about her own experience in leading these groups. She liked to envision the women's process as a journey. Along the way, she had many roles: therapist, teacher, nurturing parent. But most of all, she was a guide. For the women, that meant they didn't have to make the journey alone.

It was in being witness to the changes in these women that Marti had grown to love her job. She found helping them develop insight into themselves to be a thrilling experience. Watching this evolve into increasingly supportive relationships with their families, friends, and coworkers was rewarding to the therapist. As she had so often observed, it was in this way that the real Self within each individual felt safe to emerge. All that began to happen within the first few weeks. And as it did, the partnership among the group members deepened, causing group to become Group! Here she was, Marti thought, about to watch it happen all over again. Smiling, she turned the knob, swung the door wide, and said, "Hello."

* * * * * *

In the brief moment between opening the door and welcoming the women, Marti had time to see how the five women sitting in her waiting room were relating to one another. Each group was so different. Some started their first meeting with everyone acting like old friends. This time, however, everyone had their eyes firmly on the pages of magazines in their laps. At the sound of her voice, those five sets of eyes lifted. Some contained a look of expectancy. But it cloaked, Marti knew, considerable anxiety. "I'm so glad you're all here," she said. "Come on in and we'll get started."

First to rise was Margaret. Having met with each of these women in private sessions after they'd signed up, Marti knew that the oldest had been referred to the program by her psychiatrist. Maybe knowing what to expect is why Margaret seemed more relaxed than the others. Margaret, Marti recalled, was a housewife. Next to rise was Julie, her long hair pulled back into a ponytail. She was a librarian whose glasses kept slipping down her nose. Then came Emily, who, Marti remembered, was extremely personable and funny. They'd laughed a lot during their hour together. Emily's cheerful disposition certainly helped her, Marti thought, in her job as office manager for a family medical practice.

Next to get to her feet was Bobbie. Seeing her purse strap still slung over one shoulder, Marti thought she looked like someone was ready to get up and flee. She'd been right up front in their meeting about her years of failure. Seeing a strained expression on her face, Marti's practiced eye detected a reluctance in being here. Bobbie had not yet fully committed to this.

Last up was Kate, wearing another knock-out scarf and pair of exotic earrings. Strange, Marti thought, that she'd elected to read rather than get to know the others. If anyone knew how to break the ice, it was Kate. But this evening, Kate seemed tense – as if she was waiting for an invisible shoe to drop. For a first meeting, Marti thought, everything was going just fine. Beckoning, she invited them to follow her down the hall.

Gathering up their belongings, the women followed Marti single-file down a wide hallway. Third in line, Bobbie was seriously regretting not having bolted and run. Had there not been women behind her, she'd do it right now. But, trapped between strangers, she couldn't. And then Marti reached the door to the conference room. Standing aside, she motioned them forward, saying, "Please come in and take any chair you want. Then, fill out a name tag." Doing as they were bidden, everyone gave immense concentration to completing this first assignment. Even as Bobbie did, however, she wondered if she had made a mistake. What would this Marti person expect of her? How much would she be expected to reveal tonight? How many more minutes were there before they could go?

Bobbie wasn't the only person asking herself pretty much the same questions. But what was different about Bobbie was that she was so consumed with her own discomfort that she hadn't picked up on anyone else's even as she scrawled "Bobbie" on the sticky-backed name tag. Outwardly, now, Bobbie no longer gave the slightest hint of being ill-at-ease. Had an outsider entered just then, it might have appeared that of the five, only Julie was uncomfortable. It just wasn't true. Instead, each of these women were masters at hiding their feelings.

First to finish, Margaret took time to look over her surroundings. She was pleased to find the conference room was as comfortable as it was beautiful. While Margaret and the others surveyed their surroundings, Bobbie was still caught up in the worried confines of her mind. The only attention she'd given to her physical comfort was that she felt faintly constricted. Was she going to be expected to tell strangers how much she weighed? And what else would they want to know about her? Vowing that if she was asked, she would give as little information as humanly possible. That was the moment that Emily took to whisper to Marti, "You have a very pretty office!" Startled into looking up, Bobbie saw everyone nodding in agreement. Camilla would agree, too, Bobbie thought. Did that mean that she was trapped with a bunch of women who had nothing more on their minds than decorating?

This was a sensitive issue with Bobbie. Her mother and Melanie were always after her to do something about her condo. Already in it a year, Bobbie still had boxes in her rooms. She'd tried to shut Camilla and Melanie up by tacking swatches of fabric to the walls, but it hadn't worked. They just didn't understand that after her shift she was too tired to do anything more than get into her car, steer it through a drive-through to pick up dinner, and drive home. On the nights that Garth was home, she eliminated the trip to the drive-through because he had dinner ready when she got home. Fortunately, he didn't expect her to entertain him with stories of what went on at the hospital; he was happy enough talking about his own day. By then, her fatigue was so complete that it precluded any activity but sleep. She'd begun wondering lately if that was the reason Garth had not asked her to marry him. It didn't make it any easier to have her mother and sister ask her when she and Garth were getting married. Then, jerking her thoughts away from that, she looked up at Marti. When were they going to get started? And then, seeing that everyone was ready, Marti did.

"I want to welcome each of you to the first meeting of Phase One," she said. "As you know, I'm a clinical psychologist, and I've been leading these groups for over five years. I am very excited about this group and our first meeting tonight. Each time I start a new group, I am reminded of all the women in former groups, and I think of all the wonderful changes they made in themselves." Marti saw the expressions on their faces. "Like all of you," she said, "they came to their first meeting of Phase One filled with anticipation and questions such as: Am I doing the right thing? Will this program really help me to lose weight?" Uncomfortable with the therapist's insight, Bobbie wondered how Marti had known what she was thinking. But Marti was continuing, "Starting tonight, you will find that this program is very different from anything you have tried before. And that's because the program was designed to help each of you discover the real reasons why you eat when you're not physically hungry." She paused and then added, "I hope you noticed that I haven't mentioned anything about food so far. With this program, we will not be giving you a list of foods you can eat, and foods you cannot eat. Additionally, you will not be expected to keep track of everything you eat." Seeing relief cross their faces, she continued.

"Our program does not judge your success or failure on just the amount of weight you lose. Weight loss is the reason you are all here, and it is a very important reason. But with this program, we make another distinction. We focus on permanent weight loss. We want you to be able to keep off all the weight that you will be losing. Sometimes this happens more slowly than you expect because we are so used to quick weight loss. This is not a quick-weight loss program. Commercial diets, and some medical diets as well, emphasize the speed with which people lose weight on their special liquids or food. They are not interested in maintaining weight loss, so they don't give you anything other than their magical food. Then, when you start eating regular food again, the weight creeps right back on. Losing weight and keeping it off is not simple. Actually, it's a very complicated process!"

Marti looked at each person and saw that she had their undivided attention. "We have found that permanent weight loss cannot be achieved without looking at all levels of awareness: behaviors, thoughts, feelings, and the physical reactions," she continued. "Before we go any further, I'd like for each of you to introduce yourselves and tell us a little about your family, job, and diet experiences. Who would like to start?"

Here we go, Bobbie thought, and I'm not going first! She consciously cast her eyes downward. Someone else could volunteer! Relieved to hear Margaret say she'd go first, Bobbie went back to agonizing over what she should, and should not, say when her turn came.

Smiling pleasantly, Margaret began. "I've been married for over 30 years. We got married while I was still in college and, because my husband is very traditional, I haven't worked since my youngest son was born." Just like her mother, Bobbie thought. But it would drive her nuts to stay at home and not work. Among the others, there was some surprise. Margaret didn't look old enough to be married that long.

Margaret went on to say that her husband was a corporate attorney. Smiling, she explained that she had been perfectly happy staying home to keep house after their two sons were born. Her oldest son, she said, was single, her youngest divorced. "But, before his marriage ended," she said, "he gave me the most wonderful granddaughter in the world." Her eyes twinkled here, letting everyone know just how much she loved the child. "And with Donnie back home with us, now, I get to take care of Devon three weekends a month." Then it was time to address the issue that had brought her here tonight.

"As for my weight," Margaret said, her happy countenance fading, "I was thin as a rail as a young child, just like Devon. Then I started gaining weight around the age of seven or eight and remained chubby until after high school. I went through a thin period from college to the birth of my first son," she said, all hint of her former happiness gone, "I gained more weight during my second pregnancy and no matter what I did, I couldn't get rid of it. But, for years after, I pretty much weighed the same. Then, over the past two years, I've put on another 50 pounds." Now, her expression revealed a sense of desperation. Eyebrows knotting together, she said, "Here I am at an all-time high, and I don't know what to do about it. I tried dieting, but it didn't work. I can't live in a body that looks like this!" To herself, Margaret was wondering if she should tell them about the abuse she'd suffered as a child. Maybe, there was a connection between it and her weight. Fear of revealing too much kept her from mentioning it. "As for my diet history, I'd like to say that I'm tired of listening to so-called weight loss experts who make promises they can't keep! Their diets just don't work for me anymore." She paused for a moment, so Marti decided to insert a comment.

"You're right," she said. "Those experts try to convince us that they know more about our bodies than we do. In doing that, they assume power over what we choose to eat, and how much we choose to eat. In this program, we believe differently because we know that you can trust your body to know what's best for it!" Seeing the shock on their faces, she said, "I know that it's hard to believe, but after years of being told what and how much to eat, your head becomes disconnected from your body. When you don't have communication with your body, it's hard to know when you're hungry or when you're full, or anything else your body might need. DIETLESS helps you reconnect your body with your mind, which allows you to listen to your body's cues. When you listen, you begin to discover just how much you can trust your body to tell you exactly what it needs or wants." Having said this, Marti looked around for comments. Eagerly, Emily agreed. "What gets me," she said, "are those super-young, super-thin, diet counselors."

"Have any of you been in a program where you had to wear a leather piggy nose all evening because you hadn't lost any weight that week?" asked Margaret.

"You're kidding!" Bobbie said, startled into speaking out loud. At least she'd been spared that! Then, seeing Bobbie's signal that her outburst was the only thing she had to say on the matter, Margaret finished up by saying, "Well, I have, only it didn't help me one bit. I just went away feeling ashamed of myself." Marti underscored Margaret's statement. "Humiliation never promotes positive change," she said. Making eye contact with each one of them, she asked, "When you feel bad, what do you do?"

"Eat!" said Emily, answering for everyone. Then, seeing that Margaret was finished, she said, "I'll go next." Emily's story differed significantly from Margaret's. She had a boy who was 8, and a girl, 12. Her husband was a computer programmer, she had worked since graduating from college, and she'd been on diets since the age of four. The last shocked everyone. Four? "I was chubby at birth," Emily explained. "From what I've been told, I came out of the womb hungry. And I've been," she confessed, "hungry ever since!"

Kate was next. She told them that she and her husband owned a contracting business, that her children were grown, and that she has had a weight problem for most of her adult life. "It's gotten to where I don't know which way to turn," she said. "In the past eight years, I've gained nearly a hundred pounds. I feel like I should put a lock and key on the refrigerator and cupboards!" Everyone knew just how Kate felt.

Only Bobbie and Julie were left, and both were reluctant to speak up. Torn between the anxiety of speaking and the anxiety of more waiting and being the last to speak, Julie raised her hand. "I'm Julie," she said, her voice wobbling a little. "I've been married for nine years, and have a two-year-old son, and a four-year-old daughter."

And then, trying to hurry, she said, "I'm a librarian for a local school district. As for my diet history…" Here she hesitated. Struggling to say the right thing and no more, she said, "As a child, I guess my weight was normal. I was a little heavy when I got married, but I've been gaining ever since. I've gone on the same diets as everyone else and none of them have worked. I just keep gaining more and more weight." Julie sighed with relief. It was over. Of all of them so far, Julie was far and away the most uncomfortable in talking about herself. Marti made a mental note that Julie was consciously or unconsciously trying not to stand out. Having attention focused on her seemed difficult for her, for some reason. Now, everyone's eyes turned to Bobbie.

Earlier, when Marti talked about trusting your body, Bobbie had thought, Yeah, like she was going to trust something that had done nothing but betray her all her life! And how could a program based upon self-trust be realistic? On the other hand, she had to admit, programs based upon NOT trusting oneself certainly hadn't worked. So, now that her turn was here, Bobbie had gone from being uneasy to terror-stricken.

Used to hiding her feelings behind a mask of professionalism, Bobbie did what she always did: she pushed her feelings back and engaged her mind. Leaning forward, she prepared to speak and was startled to see that the others had all of their attention focused on her. She smiled. Surprisingly, everyone smiled back. Then she remembered that this was an informal situation. Hoping to say only the right things, she introduced herself. Using only her first name, she explained that she was a physician in the emergency room at a teaching hospital. Too intent upon her own performance, she didn't pick up the reaction to this announcement. So she went on with, "I'm not married. But I have a boyfriend, and we've been together for nearly two and a half years." To Bobbie's left, Kate was impressed. With a doctor in the group, maybe there's something to this program after all, she thought.

Emily wasn't as optimistic as Kate. What could she have in common with a doctor? Curious, now, she moved slightly forward in her seat. From there, she had a better look at Bobbie, and that's when she saw the lines in the doctor's face, and the dark shadows under her eyes. She must have been on call last night, thought Emily. Julie, too, was surprised to have a doctor in their midst. Thinking that doctors were all rich, Julie remembered that Bobbie was the one who arrived in that old van. But, then, not wanting to miss what Bobbie was saying, Julie went back to listening.

"I've been on diets since I was 14, but as you can see, they haven't worked for me either!" Bobbie said, safely answering the basic questions they'd been assigned. But something inside her forced her to add, "Which doesn't make sense because I'm good about doing exactly what I'm supposed to do." Having said that, she found herself saying even more. "Like you were saying earlier," she said, looking at Marti, "how do I know that this is going to work?"

Marti acknowledged what had been said. "Any time we are about to try something completely new, it's understandable that we have fears and doubts," she said. "What I can tell you is that everyone who's gone through this program started out feeling as you do. But by the time they were finished, they were not only losing weight, but they had also acquired the tools to continue losing and then maintain it. Along the way, each of them created a lifestyle to support the changes they had made." Bobbie was disappointed that she wasn't given a guarantee, but she hid her feelings behind a smile and a nod as Marti continued talking. "Thank you for all your introductions," she said. "Now, let's get started with the first tool to help you lose weight and keep it off. We call it TEAM eating." Going on, she explained that often, eating is done unconsciously and unconscious eating leads to weight gain. "A good example of this is – let's say that you have a bag of Hershey's kisses. You open the bag and the next thing you know, there's a big pile of silver wrappers, and only five kisses are left. Has this happened to you?" Everyone had to laugh. A few even nodded. Marti laughed, too, thinking what a great group this was. "TEAM eating," she explained, "is the acronym we use to help you identify the different kinds of unconscious eating."

Continuing, Marti said, "With conscious eating, you can enjoy what you are eating because you are aware of the taste, texture, aroma, and everything else, and you are only eating when you are physically hungry. You are aware of when your body is full or satisfied and you stop. With conscious eating, you lose weight and keep it off." Everyone looked a little stunned. Knowing that it was a lot of information, Marti said, "All of this is new, I know, but you've all eaten consciously before – we all have. When we were babies we ate only when we were hungry, and no one could make you eat past the point where you were satisfied. But as we grew, developed, and became part of family and society, we had to live by someone else's schedules, rules, and expectations. Over time, this has distracted us from the real reason we need to eat, which is to nourish and replenish those nutrients our bodies must have to survive."

Turning to the board behind her, Marti wrote the word "TEAM" vertically on the board.

T

E

A

M

With that finished, she drew an equal sign after the T, then the word "Time." Turning back to them, she pointed to the word and said, "What we mean by 'time' is eating according to the clock and not necessarily when you are physically hungry." Seeing that everyone was with her, Marti returned to the board and wrote an equal sign next to the E, then the word "Emotion." "This is when we eat in response to feelings, like anger, frustration, or boredom." Hearing a slight hum of agreement, Marti knew they were all familiar with that one. So she asked, "How many of you have eaten after having a fight with someone? Who has eaten to celebrate something? Who thinks of eating as a reward after a hard day's work?" Every hand shot up on the first question, and remained in the air for the others as well. "Guilty as charged," Kate joked. Everyone chuckled.

"We're all guilty of this," Marti said. "Human beings are very social, and part of getting together usually involves food. Graduations, for example, and weddings, funerals, holidays, and birthdays. There are many feelings attached to these events and, for many of us, food was the only way we had to deal with our feelings. So, it's hard because most of our celebrations center around food."

Proceeding on to the next letter, Marti wrote "Amount." "An example of that kind of unconscious eating is when you go to a restaurant, order your food, and, when it's placed before you, you eat everything on the plate. You have no idea if your body needed more, or less, food. You eat it because it's there. It's important to consider whether you might have wanted more food in different proportions. Did your mother ever say something like 'You should be grateful to have all this good food because there are starving children in India?'" Again, everyone chuckled. No one knew that Julie was just going along with the group. She couldn't remember her mother saying anything at mealtimes; all she could remember was that, most of the time, it was just Julie and her brother.

Kate couldn't help herself. She had to say it, "I told my mother that she could just send it to those children, but it didn't work. I had to eat it anyway." Margaret went on from there. "I got to be very good at hiding food in my napkin. It was a secret I shared with my dog."

"This," Marti said, "is another example of how unconscious eating starts. Someone else decides how much your body needs." Then she went to the last letter. "M," she said, "stands for 'Mechanical Eating,' which is when you go to a party and eat because you're expected to eat. You don't want to hurt the hostess's feelings, so you feel obliged to eat, or there's a potluck at work and you're sure everyone is watching to see that you try whatever they have prepared." Everyone nodded. "Sometimes, when you go to these parties and celebrations, you're really hungry. Other times, you aren't hungry at all. But it doesn't matter – you eat anyway." Referring back to the board where she'd written "T E A M," she asked, "Any questions?" Kate had one. She didn't quite understand, so she asked, "Would you go over Mechanical Eating again?"

"Of course," Marti replied, anxious to make it as clear as possible. "Mechanical Eating is going to a fast-food restaurant and ordering the same thing every time without asking ourselves if that is what we really want to eat. Then, automatically, we eat it all. Many times, taste hasn't entered the picture. So the food is not really enjoyed." Kate nodded, letting Marti know that it now made sense to her. Turning to the group, Marti announced, "I have one more tool for you. From this moment on, each of you will be a FOOD CRITIC."

"A food critic?" asked Emily. Marti nodded. "Starting right now, you will choose only the very best food to put into your body. That means, if you are physically hungry and decide that you want a chocolate chip cookie, go ahead and eat one. But eat the best chocolate chip cookie you can find. And if you find after one bite it isn't as good as you expected, don't finish it." Margaret was the first to respond. "What do we do with it if we don't like it?"

"Throw it away," Marti replied.

Anxiety filled the air. Emily was the first to say, "Isn't that wasting food?" Marti nodded. "It probably feels that way," she admitted. "But to finish a bag of cookies that you don't like just because they would be wasted isn't a good enough reason for you to eat them. If you can't throw it away, give the food to a friend, your kids, or your pets." Hesitantly, Julie asked, "What will our husbands and children think if they see us throwing food away?"

Then Marti said something that no one had ever said to them before. "It doesn't matter what anyone else thinks," she said. "The only thing that matters is that you deserve to eat only the best."

Deserve? They deserved the best? Somewhere deep down inside, each woman wanted to believe that this was true. Feeling overwhelmed, Kate asked, "How are we going to remember all this?"

"We have something here that is going to help," replied Marti, as she carried a stack of purse-sized notebooks to the table. "These are your workbooks," she said. "Your first assignment is inside."

The first to receive hers, Kate was pleased to see that the notebook had a plain cover. She wasn't carrying anything around that advertised her participation in a weight-loss program! Bobbie was glad about that, too. She was equally pleased to see that the notebook was arranged just like the best business organizers, with plenty of room to keep track of appointments and dates. And, although Julie would not have said anything aloud, she liked the size because it was small enough to fit in her purse and big enough to keep everything together.

Emily idly leafed through the first week's assignment. For each day, there were two pages. On one side was space for listing appointments and things to do. On the other was a journal. Look, she thought, every day has a different question. Then she noticed the phrase, *Eat what you really want when you are hungry, and stop when you are full.* They must really want us to remember this, she thought, because it's on every single page. But how was this going to help them lose weight? Well, she might not have the answer to that, but she liked the book anyway.

Across the table, Julie was turning her pages with the delicate touch of a true book-lover. Her attention, too, was caught by the message at the top of the page. She particularly liked "Eat what you want." She was less sure about "when you are hungry, and stop when you are full." She wondered how she was ever going to know if her body felt hungry or full. Then she noticed that on each page that statement was followed by a different question, none of which looked threatening. Not so for Bobbie, who reacted to them with a flutter of worry. How was she going to be able to find time to do all this? But closer inspection reassured her that the questions were direct and straightforward, and they wouldn't demand a great deal of time.

"Each week, I will be giving you the next week's assignment, with questions centered around a new topic. This week, we are asking questions that will help you become more aware of your unconscious eating – or TEAM eating. These notebooks are for your own private use. No one is going to read them, or ask you to read from them. However, to get the most out of this program, we encourage you to answer the questions every day. Even if you haven't written down your answers, we want you to come to class and tell us what you think and feel regarding the assignment." Seeing that there were no more questions, Marti ended the meeting with a friendly, "See you next week."

First out the door, Margaret headed across the parking lot, more hopeful than she'd been in a long time. But by the time she had pulled out her keys, she returned to justifying the upcoming expense. Thank heaven their insurance would pay for 80%. Not that Bob would object to the other 20%. At least he never had. Yet she disliked having him know that she was spending money on another diet. She might fail again. On the other hand, a cheerful note in her memory reminded her, Marti had brought up some suggestions and concepts that she had never heard before. For some reason, they resonated with something deep inside her. Her mind swimming between hope and fear, Margaret decided to think about something more pleasant: her granddaughter, Devon.

Emily, having determined that she had a lot in common with Kate, walked out with her. "I really think this is going to work," Emily said. Smiling at her, Kate hid her own reservations. "Hope you're right." Then they parted, each going to her own car. Unhappily, Emily found her confidence ebbing the instant she was alone. Inside her car, she told herself that what Marti had said sounded terrific except she hadn't said how long it would take to lose the weight. Staring at the steering wheel, Emily wondered, Why can't there be a magic pill to make this happen right now?

Across the parking lot, Bobbie was already tossing everything into her car. Eager to be on her way, she slid in without noticing that her lipstick had fallen out of her purse and lay on the floor. Nor was she aware that her workbook had tumbled into the space between the seats. They only blended into the clutter already there.

Bobbie busied herself wriggling around to tug at the fabric of her pants so they wouldn't bind. Absently, she noted that they fit better than most, which meant that she didn't have to shop again for a while. That reminded her of Kate, who wore such pretty scarves. Bobbie wished she could wear pretty things like that. I wonder where she gets them, she thought. This led her to reflect that Kate and the others seemed nice enough. Bobbie turned the key and pulled forward. Entering the line of traffic, her mind switched to Garth, who was out of town. So she fell into her regular questioning: did she want a frozen dinner or fast food? The drive-through won.

While waiting to place her order on the outdoor monitor, Bobbie remembered to do as Marti had suggested: she would ask her body what it really wanted to eat. Feeling somewhat ridiculous, she whispered, "OK, body, I'm listening." Sure that she heard her body answer that it was starved, she felt no remorse in replying to the voice that emerged from the speaker. "Order, please," said the voice, and Bobbie ordered her usual: a double cheeseburger, jumbo fries, onion rings, and a large diet cola. Then, reminding herself again to order what she really wanted, she changed the diet cola to a regular cola.

Driving ahead to the pick-up window, she accepted her drink and, knowing that the rest of the order would take a few minutes, inserted her straw through the container lid and took a small sip. Remembering that she was now a food critic, she held the soda in her mouth and allowed her tastebuds to react to the liquid sweetness. It surprised her how much better the regular cola tasted. But then her food was ready and, from that point on, Bobbie lost all conscious awareness. Heading out of the parking lot, she began eating. Within a few minutes she had consumed the entire burger, half the drink, all the onion rings, and most of the fries. Because she wasn't paying attention, she missed the messages her body was sending. From force of habit, she polished off the remaining fries and the rest of the cola before reaching her freeway off-ramp.

Homeward bound, Julie was still pondering what Marti had said: TEAM eating, conscious eating, unconscious eating, becoming a food critic, and talking in front of the group. It hadn't been so awful, after all. But what was she going to say next week?

CHAPTER THREE

Emily vs Three Dozen Cookies

Week Four: Feeling Deprived Leads to Weight Gain

*M*ARTI FOUND THE WAITING ROOM filled with women's voices and scents of their perfumes and lotions. Engaged with each other, none of the four noticed that she'd opened the hallway door. It took her, "Hi," to get their attention. Looking up into her smiling face, they all smiled back. In that simple interaction it was evident how far they'd come in one short month. There were good reasons for this. For Margaret, it was finding out that she wasn't ever going to have to get weighed in group – ever. She started feeling more comfortable right away. Knowing that there weren't any sacred calorie or fat gram rules to violate made her feel even safer. She, along with Julie and Emily, now felt better about the weekly assignments, too. Ironically, the exercises had less to do with food than with being aware of it. The result was that Margaret was paying closer attention to what she ate, and trying to decide whether she liked it and whether she was getting enough.

Julie was relieved at how much easier everything was than she'd expected. Maybe that's why, she thought, she had learned so much in such a short time. That is what Julie had been hearing Emily, Margaret, and Kate say just before Marti opened the door. Had Marti not come in just then, Julie might even have joined the conversation. But now that everyone was on their way to the conference room, it was too late. Well, not everyone, because Bobbie wasn't there yet. Her tardiness to group, as it turned out, wasn't unusual. Julie wondered if Bobbie was late to everything – or just this class. Glancing over at Marti, Julie saw the therapist check her watch. They might have to start without Bobbie!

Kate, Emily, Margaret, and Julie took their usual seats, ready to start. It had been almost a month, and all had come to the same realization: no matter what happened anywhere else in their lives, they could always count on their 15 minutes of undivided attention here in group. For most, this attention had been, at first, a little uncomfortable. It was amazing, but none of them had ever experienced being heard before. But here, people really listened, without responding judgmentally or with criticism. Julie had the most fear to overcome, but just being able to say what she felt comfortable saying was in itself a big accomplishment. Everyone used their time to talk about what happened with last week's assignment. With the time left over, they brought up things that bothered them during the week. From the second week together, each had begun bringing up more personal problems, some having to do with work, others with relationships. Whatever the subject, those listening were increasingly comfortable asking questions or making suggestions. So what began as a soliloquy most often ended up as either a dialogue between two members or as a conversation in which everyone got involved. Each week, the five were getting closer to being a Group.

During their first three weeks together, the women had spent considerable time describing the struggle to relinquish their old diet rules. It was something that they had to do if they were to ever be free from all the false hopes and empty promises. The rule that refused to die was the one having to do with "good" and "bad" foods. Saying it almost like a mantra, Marti always responded with, "Food is neither good nor bad. Food is only fuel for the body!" It had gotten to the point where they all joined in when she started saying it. But even as they teased Marti, they knew it was true, intellectually, if not emotionally. And Marti always followed up with, "The only time you should use 'good or bad' as a description of your food is when you are determining how a food makes your body feel. You will have some reactions immediately, others may not occur for an hour or two. So, after you eat, does your body feel tired? Sluggish? Is your stomach upset? Did the food you ate give you diarrhea? When the answer is yes to any of these, it describes a 'bad' food. That doesn't mean that you can never eat that particular food, only that you would want to select a convenient time to eat it." The reason she urged them to do this, Marti told them, was because they deserved to feel good.

She deserved to feel good? Emily had never considered that before. But, then, she hadn't expected that simply by discussing all these things she was gaining insight into conclusions she'd drawn and assumptions she'd never before questioned. But there was something Marti said that Emily couldn't accept – that she could eat what she'd previously classified as "bad" foods without losing all of her hard-won self-control. Scared to try, Emily hadn't put her body to the trust-test yet. It was one thing, she figured, to have someone tell you that you could have faith in your body to make the right decisions. It was quite another to turn it loose around all those forbidden goodies, especially when you suspected that if you ate even a tiny bit of real ice cream, you'd max out the dairy case! Despite her difficulties with these concepts, Emily drew comfort from knowing that she was discovering a lot about herself that she had not known, not only from Marti, but from the other group members as well.

Watching the four settle in, Marti was also reviewing their month-long history together. Because each of the women was such an individual, it was expected that each of them would address an issue in their own way. That was the strength of the program – everyone could customize the program to meet their own individual needs. Margaret had been the first to notice the change in her "food thoughts." Responding to that, Marti said, "Once you begin to listen to your body and eat more consciously, your thoughts will no longer be focused on food." Maybe for Margaret, Emily thought, but not for her. She was still obsessing several times a day about what she wanted to eat, or not having enough time to eat it, or that everyone would have eaten everything before she got to it.

Julie, on the other hand, was challenged by other obstacles. It's easier for people who stay in the office all day, she told herself. But her job called for her to travel all over the district, so she never knew where she was going to be. If she hadn't been afraid of sounding like an idiot, Julie would have brought this up. But because she wanted so badly for the others to like her, she didn't dare let them know how little of the program she was understanding. So far, all she had shared was that she nibbled and snacked between meals. Marti had praised her for her growing awareness. That had made Julie feel better about things. But not good enough to take a chance on saying too much.

Marti had observed Julie's reluctance to talk about her experiences and feelings. Something, the therapist thought, or someone had taught Julie to hold back information about herself. But no matter, Marti thought, Julie would talk when she was ready. Listening to others come to common understandings would help her. One day soon, Marti trusted, after hearing how someone else's eating habits related to their familial or societal expectations, Julie would ask herself whose expectations she was trying to live up to. Who was it who had told her how she should look, how much she should weigh, what she should – and should not – eat. The reasons behind anyone's weight were very complex. Often, the answers came in the form of revelations.

Kate was having one of those right now – she just didn't know it. While removing her jacket, she found her mind returning to Ed and where he might be. He hadn't come home after work last night and didn't show up before she left for the office this morning. He hadn't shown up all day, either. Then, catching her runaway thoughts, she grew annoyed with herself. Why should she let thoughts of him intrude on her private time? Ordering herself to forget him, Kate focused on what was happening here in group.

As Marti was asking, "Who wants to go first?" Kate, who'd gone from worrying about Ed to realizing that she'd not finished the assignment, avoided opening her notebook. She was relieved when rescue arrived in the form of Bobbie, rushing in with a flurry of apologies.

"Sorry," she breathed as she flung her jacket over the back of the chair and claimed her seat. Right away, she opened her notebook. Hers, like Kate's, had several pages that were still blank. Unlike Kate, Bobbie wasn't embarrassed about it – she was furious. With herself. This was the fourth week and she had not once finished the weekly assignments. What was the matter with her, she demanded of herself. Why hadn't she taken the time to do this?

"This past week," Marti was saying, "the assignment focused on eating only the foods that you like, and making sure that they were available to you no matter where you were. So how did that go for everyone?"

Emily responded first. "I really like the cookies at this one bakery, so I went there and bought some." Suddenly reluctant to just come right out and say how many she'd purchased, Emily said, "Because Marti told us to make sure that we always had enough, I bought three dozen. Then, I took them back to the car and ate every one of them right then and there." With that said, Emily paused. Had she done the assignment right? Would Marti be mad at her? Several of the others were waiting to find out the same thing. So everyone was surprised when Marti asked, "How did that make you feel?"

"Terrific!" said Emily, so relieved that she smiled broadly.

"Did you have enough?" Marti asked.

"For the first time in my life!" Emily declared.

"How did they taste?" pursued Marti. "Did the last one taste as good as the first? What about the ones in the middle?"

Surprised by the questions, Emily had to admit that she didn't know. "I was concentrating on eating as many as I wanted," she said.

"Well," Marti observed. "Sounds like you satisfied your head – but how did your body feel? Did it enjoy the taste, the texture, and the smell?"

Again, Emily confessed that she didn't know. Then something occurred to her. More cheerfully, she said, "I guess I wasn't paying attention – but I know that I didn't get sick afterwards!"

"That," Marti said, "is a good observation." Then she led Emily into investigating her reactions further by asking, "You didn't get sick, but did your body feel good after eating the cookies?" For the third time, Emily didn't know. "I'll have to think about it," she said, her short-lived liveliness gone.

Pleased that Emily was becoming more aware, Marti wanted to encourage her to expand that awareness even further. So she said, "I have a suggestion. When you do this again, take the time to enjoy each and every bite. As you're eating your first cookie, notice what you're experiencing in your nose, your mouth, and your stomach. Do this with every cookie you eat, asking yourself how each one feels in your body. Is there an after-taste? What's the difference between having one cookie in your body and seven? How many does it take to make you feel energized, or comfortable, or sleepy… or full?" Turning to the rest of them, Marti commented, "The point, here, is that each of you should maximize each eating experience. Part of doing that is consciously enjoying everything that you eat."

Although no one would have guessed by looking at Julie, what

Marti was saying was going right over her head. She was too caught up in admiring the openness with which Emily was able to talk about all those cookies. She had been just as candid about her childhood, too. Julie couldn't imagine telling anyone that she'd been turned into a misfit by her mother, much less admitting to having gobbled down three dozen cookies in broad daylight in the middle of town. Torn between admiration and shame, Julie knew that she could never reveal anything that personal. But, as Emily continued, Julie stopped ruminating in time to hear her say, "Since I ate all the cookies, I decided to go in and buy more and bring them home. But," she said, her voice oddly flat, "my husband and kids thought they were for everyone and ate them all up."

"How did you feel about that?" Marti asked.

"Like there's never enough for me!"

Emily's response caught everyone by surprise. The tone in her voice made it hard to tell if she was angry, or hurt or what. So everyone just sat there, trying to figure it out. Margaret, who remembered what it was like to have ever-hungry children who assumed that everything in the house was theirs for the taking, said, "I think I would have been so disappointed that I'd have felt like crying." And Kate, whose children had been just like Margaret's, asked, "So what did you say when you found out the cookies were gone?" Hearing the honest concern behind these questions, Emily bit her lip. Her voice wobbling, she said, "I didn't say anything because I didn't want to be selfish."

Marti, who was about to ask the others what they thought, saw that Kate wanted to respond and told her to go ahead. "If you didn't say anything, what did you do?" Her face flushing, Emily replied, "I panicked!" She stopped there, suddenly unable to say one more thing. Knowing the importance of having Emily give voice to her feelings, Marti said, "What did you do with that feeling?"

Emily hesitated. How honest should she be? It would be too embarrassing to admit what she had done – that she waited until everyone was asleep, then ate every one of the brownies she'd baked for the kids' lunches. Her struggles to decide what she was going to say were clearly visible to the others. Again, Kate spoke up. "I would have eaten something!" she said. Surprised, Emily looked around and found everyone nodding, telling her that what she'd done was not surprising to any of them. So she confessed, "I ate my children's brownies," she said. "But I regretted it because I felt sick afterward!" Wanting the others to see that Emily had eaten in response to a feeling, Marti said, "So you panicked, and the only thing you could do to take care of that feeling was to eat brownies." When Emily nodded, Marti said, "Let's look at some of the other choices you might want to make next time." And she turned to the others to see what suggestions they might have.

Throughout the discussion, Bobbie wanted to ask why Emily hadn't just gone out and bought more cookies. Now, she asked that. "I thought about it," Emily admitted. "But what good would it do? When my family sees them, they'll just assume that I bought more for them and I'll be right back where I started – with no cookies for me!"

Wanting to help Emily identify how she'd felt when her food was unexpectedly not there, Marti said, "What most women feel when they find their food gone or denied to them is deprivation. And that's followed by panic." Heads around the table nodded. "It doesn't matter if someone else eats it all up, or tells you that you can't have it, your food is gone! That sets you up to binge. Feeling deprived causes you to eat the cookies even when your body is not physically hungry, and then the feelings of desperation and panic stop. But all you've done is give yourself a temporary respite from deprivation. An hour later, seeing the empty cookie bag makes you feel guilty, which triggers the desperation all over again. That's how you continue the cycle of eating to push down feelings – and that, of course, leads to weight gain."

Looking around the table, Marti saw that everyone understood all too well. So she continued, "What we need to relearn is that food is plentiful. That's why we want you to make sure that from now on you have more than enough of your favorite foods on hand. That means if you normally buy three bags of cookies, we want you to buy six."

"Six? Why so many?" protested Margaret. Marti was ready to answer that. "Part of it is visual," she said. "Seeing that you have more than enough is reassuring. It lets you know that you can have some whenever you want. So, what do you do when it's gone?" Not waiting for them to answer, Marti said, "Go get some more." That made sense, everyone agreed.

"Any time we don't have what we want, we have the power to get it," Marti said. "So when you run low of your favorite things, or you want something that you don't have, you can go out and do something about it. In this way, you show yourself that you're not helpless, but rather perfectly capable of providing whatever your body needs and wants."

The word "helpless" hit a chord in Emily. It's exactly how she'd felt when she was a child and her mother said, "No, no, Emily, you can't have that; it'll make you fat. Here, take this instead." What "this" usually turned out to be were a few of those tasteless animal crackers from the circus train box. She hated those animals, not only because they tasted like sand but also because no one else wanted to eat them. She had no choice.

Seeing Emily drift away, Marti brought her back with, "Emily, what's going on inside of you right now?" Startled, Emily thought a minute, then said, "The word 'helpless' started me thinking. Until I went away to college, my mother controlled everything I ate. When my brother and sisters got mashed potatoes, I got a boiled one – plain, with no butter or margarine. I could never have cake at birthday parties, I couldn't have regular desserts at home." Then, not wanting them to think that her mother was some sort of monster, she added, "Mom said she did it for my own good." Hearing that,

Margaret nearly gasped out loud. For Emily's own good? What kind of a mother would do that to a child? But Emily was continuing

"You see, Mom was right all along. When I got to college, I lived in a dorm where everything was served cafeteria-style. With no one to stop me, I ate everything. And I didn't stop until that summer when I went home. When my mother saw how much weight I'd gained, she gave me that look of total disappointment. I wanted the earth to open up and swallow me. So, that summer, I put myself on a diet – one that's never ended. I learned my lesson – the only things keeping me from gaining even more weight are foods that are low fat, calorie-free, or sugar-free."

"Do you like diet food?" asked Marti. Bobbie was right behind her with, "Do you eat regular food, too?" Emily answered Bobbie first. "Not very often!" she said. Then, after a short pause, she added, "Sometimes, I just want to eat something else. You know, real food. So I sneak some."

It was so shocking to Margaret that anyone would choose to eat nothing but diet foods that she had to ask, "What do you do about meals, like dinner? Don't you eat with the family?"

"Well, we all eat together," Emily replied, "but I stick pretty much to salads and cooked vegetables."

Margaret wanted more clarification and asked, "Are you saying that you have your food and your family has theirs?" Emily nodded. "Yes!" she said.

"Well," said Marti, "I can understand that. Growing up, you got the message that you couldn't have the same food as anyone else."

"That's right," Emily affirmed. "I'm used to eating something different from everyone else. Besides, whenever I eat their food, I always gain weight. And with my family, who knows what you'll find in the refrigerator or cupboards. So, if I have a craving for something, I've learned to make extra because the next time I want some, it probably won't be there." Marti, knowing that this was the time to sum everything up, said, "So, it appears that diet food serves a couple of purposes in your life." Wanting to know what they might be, Emily tipped her head to let Marti know that she was paying close attention.

"Diet food gives you some sense of control over your weight," Marti said. "It also gives you a feeling of security. Knowing that your food is always there and no one else wants it is comforting. But it would be interesting to know what happens to you while you are eating." Marti then asked two more questions. "Do you feel satisfied when you're eating diet food? Do diet foods help you to lose weight?" While Emily was forming her answers, Julie suddenly saw what Marti was getting at. Thrilled, she wanted to speak up and say, "But if you don't like it, it's not worth eating!" She didn't, of course.

At the same time, Bobbie was noting that this was the first time Marti had asked those particular questions. So, Bobbie wondered, did Emily lose weight eating little more than diet food? Apparently not, because Emily's answer, when it came, was "No, I'm not satisfied! And it doesn't matter how much or little I eat of anything, I've reached a point where I can't lose weight anymore. And I don't know if I really like it. Most diet food that I've tried has no flavor."

Emily continued, "I just know that it's the only safe food for me to eat. Except, something always happens and I can't help myself. I have to have something sweet. So, hating myself for doing it, I go out and buy cookies, or cinnamon rolls, or something." Having said that much, Emily felt unable to keep from telling more. "During the day, that means that I have to buy and eat it in my car during a lunch break or a run to the bank." She paused there, afraid to tell them that she did the same kind of thing late at night. She'd wait until everyone was asleep, then sneak out of bed and raid the refrigerator, or the kids' snacks. Ashamed by this, Emily decided not to tell and was relieved that Marti had turned to the others to include them in what she was saying. "What Emily says is significant. When we eat foods that don't satisfy us, we start looking around for something that will give us the taste or texture we are longing for. During

47

the searching process, we end up eating far more than our body really wants. When we finally find it, we eat that food, too. Eating food that we don't want, then eating the food that we really wanted, is called double eating and that leads to weight gain."

Until now, Kate had listened to everything and even spoke up a few times. But her mind kept asking what she was doing here. Her marriage was falling apart and she was wasting time in another weight loss program. What was she, crazy? Then she heard Marti proposing double eating as a major reason for gaining weight. That rang true, and Kate had to enter the discussion. "You mean," she inquired, "if we eat peanut butter cookies all day because that is what we really want, we'll lose weight?" Margaret, equally intrigued, added, "Or a sandwich instead of fat-free cottage cheese?"

Pleased at Kate's reawakened interest, Marti grinned and said, "Yes!" From the redhead's reaction, Marti saw how badly Kate wanted to believe this. Looking around, Marti saw that this was true of everyone. So she said, "The key is to eat the peanut butter cookie or sandwich only when you're physically hungry – and to stop eating when you're full. Over time, this kind of conscious eating helps you lose weight and keep the pounds off." Emily raised her hand. "Isn't it selfish to want to keep them for myself?" she asked. Marti's answer surprised her. "You have every right to keep things just for yourself!" Silence fell over the group, telling Marti what she suspected; these women felt no sense of ownership for themselves as individuals. It made sense, considering that girls were taught from birth that nice girls share, ideal wives accommodate, and good mothers sacrifice. So it stood to reason that the five women sitting around her conference table found it difficult to accept that they didn't have to subordinate their own desires to those of others. So Marti said again, "There is nothing selfish in keeping some favorite foods just for yourself!" Julie, obedient daughter, accommodating wife, and dedicated mother, was so rattled by this that she took her glasses off and began cleaning them. She was even more uncomfort-

able at Marti's next statement. "You will be learning to set boundaries and limits which will protect the things that are important to
you."

Margaret wasn't at all sure what Marti meant by this, but she
knew where her familial duties were. Firmly, she said, "I've always
believed that what was mine belonged to my husband and sons, too,
and sharing is part of being a family!" Marti agreed. "Of course," she
said. "sharing is part of the normal give and take of family life. But
when you share everything that's yours with your family, there is
nothing left for you. That's what leads to feeling deprived. So, what
we're aiming for is a healthy balance – some things are shared, some
are mine – and that includes food!"

Following closely now, Kate agreed. She made a suggestion, too.
"Emily, what I did with my boys was to declare that a certain cabinet
belonged to me. Inside, I kept my good scissors, glue, and other
things I didn't want them messing with. They knew that they
weren't to go in there without my permission." Listening to a few
other suggestions, Emily thought to herself that she liked Kate's idea
the best. She'd try that, she decided. Thanking everyone, she said
that she was finished.

Julie went back to worrying. Would Marti expect her to go next?
Hoping that no one was looking, Julie squirmed in her chair. How
could she tell Marti and the others what had happened when she
went to store the extra stash of her favorite food – caramelized pop-
corn and nuts? She didn't want Tom or the kids to find it, so she
couldn't put it anywhere in the kitchen. Most of the closets were too
hard for her to get into so, with no other choice available, she'd
stuck her stockpile in the bathroom closet, behind the toilet paper.
And wouldn't you know – Tom had gone in there for soap and
found them. Coming to her with the cans in his hand, he asked,
"Where'd these come from?" Not knowing how to explain, she'd
mumbled that she didn't know. Then, swiftly changing the subject
to his latest computer program, she had taken the cans from his

hands and put them on the counter. Caught up in describing his program, Tom hadn't asked any more questions. Julie wasn't sure that she could tell the group any of this, so she was grateful when Kate volunteered to go next.

Kate didn't want to admit that she hadn't done the whole assignment, but she wanted to get her confession out of the way. "I bought the food, but I didn't write anything in my notebook!" she said. Marti, recognizing that Kate's reluctance to do this week's assignment needed investigating, proceeded gently. What needed to be done when this occurred was a step-by-step questioning that guided the person into understanding why she hadn't completed her homework.

"There is no right or wrong way to do the homework," Marti said. "Sometimes when women find it difficult to do, there might be something going on that's important to understand." Relieved that she hadn't been embarrassed or yelled at in front of the others, Kate replied, "I don't know why I didn't get it done!"

Marti smiled at Kate. "Do you ever wonder what happened to that little girl you used to be? The one you can still see in family pictures?" Kate frowned. Where was Marti going with this? Knowing that the others were wondering, too, Marti continued. "She didn't go away," she said. "Each of us has that little girl inside of us. She takes care of our feelings, hopes, wishes, and dreams. But for many women," Marti said, "this feeling-part is hidden – tucked away – out of their everyday awareness. But that doesn't stop the little girl from feeling." Kate was obviously bothered by Marti's explanation. "I like to think of myself as an adult," she said. Marti nodded.

"There is another part of us inside that is the adult. The adult is the thinking part of us. She makes decisions, gets us where we need to go, balances the checkbook, and takes care of everyone else. She isn't deliberately ignoring the little girl – she's just lost touch with her. So, when the adult gets too busy and then says 'I have one more thing to do,' the little girl rebels. Most of the time, our adult isn't even aware of what's going on with that feeling part of herself."

Kate thought about this for a minute, then said, "Maybe I was rebelling. Ed was out of town last week and I had to work extra hours. By the time I got home I was so tired that the thought of writing in my journal didn't even enter my mind."

"Perhaps," Marti said, "what happened last week is that your adult was very busy taking care of everyone else. So busy that, at the end of the day, when you had time for yourself, all you felt like doing was nothing. To do something for yourself, like your journal, made your little girl say…." Marti waited for Kate to finish the sentence, and she did. "I'm tired. I want to rest. I want to go play and have fun. I don't want to do this!"

"So," Marti said, "the reason for not completing your assignment is not because you're lazy or bad. It's because other things came first, leaving you no time or energy to do what you needed to do for yourself." Marti paused to glance around the table. Everyone was paying close attention. Good, she thought, now for the food connection. Aloud, she asked what had become an infamous question. "I wonder how food fits into this?"

Kate thought about this for a minute. "All I know," she said, "is that I get awfully hungry late at night."

"Is it a physical hunger?" Marti asked.

"I can't say that it is," said Kate. "It just comes over me that I have to have potato chips and dip. I did go out and buy four bags of them, and the sour cream and onion mix to make four big helpings of dip."

"So what happened?" Emily wanted to know.

"Surprisingly enough," Kate said, "there's still some left."

"Is that unusual?" asked Marti. Laughing, Kate said, "It sure is. Before, if it was available, I ate every bit!"

Marti smiled. "So," she said, "when you knew that there was more than enough, you didn't eat as much!" Looking around the table, she added, "Kate didn't lose control just because her favorite food was available. Having more than enough gave her the choice to eat it all up – or not." Kate hadn't looked at it that way. Now, she smiled as Marti continued. "The next question is – did you eat the chips and dip only when you were hungry?"

Kate's smile disappeared. "I knew you were going to ask me that," she sighed. "So I thought about an answer on the drive over here and – no – I couldn't possibly have been hungry because I'd had a full dinner just a couple of hours earlier. It's just that I get this overpowering urge to eat again later on."

"Have you always had this urge, or did it just start?" asked Marti.

Thinking back, Kate said, "It started about eight years ago – right after we moved into our new house." Consciously, she made the decision not to mention what had happened with her friend Jody about a year earlier, or she'd have to explain about her suspicions about Jody and Ed. So Kate left all that out, saying, "Ed doesn't like any of our neighbors. He says that he hasn't got anything in common with them. He complains about their foreign cars and our house. Given the choice, he'd go back to the old one, even though it was small, dark, and crowded. He wouldn't have moved at all if our tax advisor hadn't said we needed the write-off. Besides, he's gone most of the time, so I don't know why he complains so much."

"Are you saying that you're alone a lot at night?" asked Margaret, knowing what it was like with Bob away so much. "Yes," Kate replied, trying to keep a note of bitterness from her voice. Marti followed that with, "Well, if the chips and dip aren't serving a physical need, what is there about night that makes you feel that you need them?" Kate had no immediate answer. A few seconds later, she said, "I work hard all day, and food is the only thing I have to look forward to. It's like a reward."

Hearing this, Marti thought that Kate had a number of hungers that she was trying to satisfy with food: loneliness, working too hard, lack of fun, and marital problems. As Marti was making her mental notes, Bobbie spoke up. "What Kate says is true – when we work hard, food is the only thing we have to look forward to."

"So, sometimes," Marti said, repeating this, "the only thing you have to look forward to is food. That means that you eat whether you're hungry or not. And that leads to weight gain, which ultimately makes you feel bad about yourself!" Glumly, everyone agreed. Marti went on. "So the reward isn't really a reward because it doesn't work to make you feel better." Again, everyone nodded. And Marti said, "It's scary to acknowledge that there are things in our lives that just aren't working, whether at work or home. But you know, writing about those things in your journal lets you inspect not only the situation, but your deepest feelings about it as well. Once you acknowledge your feelings, you can find other ways to take care of them." What Marti was saying made a lot of sense and Kate, for one, tucked it away to think about later. Now, however, it was still her turn.

"It was a busy week," Kate continued. "With Ed gone, I ended up having to do two jobs – his and mine! But I'm glad he's gone after what he did last weekend." And she went on to describe their annual employee barbecue.

"I'd really worked hard on planning this party," Kate said, "because I wanted the people who work for us, and their spouses, to know how much we value them. Saturday, Elite Caterers came out and prepared this beautiful buffet. Well," she sighed, "Ed started drinking around noon, and that made me really nervous because I didn't know what he would do. Then, just as the band took an intermission and everyone was lining up at the buffet, I heard Ed's voice rising above everyone else's. He was saying something inexcusably vulgar about me. He thought he was being funny. I just wanted to die."

Devastated for her friend, Emily all but whispered, "What did you do?"

Her voice letting them know how miserable she'd felt, said, "What I always do: I smiled and pretended like nothing happened"

Bobbie, knowing how this must have hurt, said, "How embarrassing for you." And Emily said, "Your husband had no right to talk about you like that." Margaret was quick to agree. "Emily's right; you don't deserve to be treated that way!"

Sitting there, hearing the Group's indignation and feeling their outrage, Kate felt something within her begin to loosen. Although she could not at that moment have verbalized what that something was, she could feel its sharp edges giving way. With that release, came tears. Slowly, at first, and startling herself more than anyone else, the tears began sliding down her cheeks. Who could have imagined how much these women would come to mean to her!

Watching Kate cry, Emily wanted desperately to lean over and put her arm around Kate's shoulders in an attempt to comfort her. But Emily didn't know whether this would help or hinder what Kate was going through. So it was Marti who responded first. "It's really hard to be so conscious of what's going on, and I'm really proud that you've been able to sit with those feelings tonight." Then Marti allowed several moments to pass so that everyone could empathize with Kate's pain. When Kate's body language indicated that she was finished, Marti wrapped everything up by saying, "It's really difficult that, as you become aware of the connection between your feelings and food, the first thing that comes up is pain. It takes a lot of courage to work through that." Then she asked who wanted to go next.

Knowing that no evasion was possible, Bobbie said, "I can understand how Kate felt admitting that she hadn't done the entire assignment." Looking directly at Marti, she went on with, "You explained that Kate's little girl was in rebellion – well, I guess I'm wondering if there is something inside of me that's rebelling, too. I work 12-hour shifts. Sometimes, I take extra hours to make more money. So there's no time for anything else."

Identifying with that, Kate asked if Bobbie ever had time to relax. That caught Bobbie by surprise, and she had to admit that she didn't. Then, embarrassed, Bobbie explained, "I haven't had any extra time in so long that I wouldn't know what to do with it if I had it!"

Not about to let that go by, Marti commented, "It sounds like, even if you had time, you'd be lost trying to figure out what to do." When Bobbie admitted that this was true, Marti asked, "How do you see your work schedule affecting your eating?" Wondering how Marti had gotten from one thing to another, Bobbie was surprised into telling the unadulterated truth. "I'd love to be able to sit down and eat my meals, but I can't because I don't have time. That's why I always eat on the run."

"Mmmmm," Marti said. "What is it like for your little girl to always be so rushed that she can't sit down and enjoy a meal?" And that's when Bobbie balked.

"I'm having a hard time accepting the idea of a little girl," she said. "I just can't picture one inside of me." Although Marti did not say it, she was wondering if Bobbie had a need to hide and protect her little girl – even from herself. Aloud, Marti said, "Many women have trouble visualizing the small child inside of them. Sometimes it's helpful to just call it 'the feeling' part of you." When Marti saw that the changed wording suited Bobbie just fine, she said, "It makes sense that the feeling part of you wanted to rebel because you so rarely have time for yourself," she said. "Adding one more thing for you to do, like your journal, probably stirs up a lot of feelings. Your job and your life are so crowded with have-to's for others that there's no room for the things you need and want. This can very easily lead to feelings of deprivation." Looking directly into Bobbie's eyes, she said, "Bobbie, you deserve more than you give yourself." Then, bringing it back to food, Marti said to Bobbie, "And at meal-time, you and your body deserve to enjoy what you're eating!"

Bobbie would liked to have felt some response to Marti's statement, but she couldn't. Mainly because she couldn't envision ever having enough time to enjoy much of anything. However, it made her feel good to hear Marti say that she "deserved" it. No one had ever even hinted at that before. Uplifted, Bobbie said, "Well, I did do one thing this week, I tried to identify which candy bar is my favorite by buying a couple dozen different kinds. But then Garth opened the drawer where I'd put them and said, 'What are these?'" Julie felt her ears prick up. So, she thought, it happened to Bobbie, too. But it was Emily who spoke. "What did you do?" she asked, and Bobbie said, "I was so shocked and embarrassed that he found out what I was doing that I acted like I'd suddenly remembered a phone call and left the room." Turning to Marti, she asked, "What should I have said?"

Instead of answering the question directly, Marti opened it up to the Group. "It's an awful feeling to be so exposed and not be able to protect yourself. What could Bobbie say if it happens again?"

Kate had the first response. "I don't know if I'd actually say this to anyone," she said, "but I'd want to say – 'Get the hell out of my drawer!'" An explosion of laughter rewarded this straightforward approach. Marti had to admit that it would sure get the message to Garth that he had invaded Bobbie's territory – her emotional as well as physical territory. Then she asked for more suggestions. When there weren't any, Marti said, "How about saying something like, 'Those are my candy bars. You can have one, but you need to ask me first!'" Bobbie wasn't so sure. "Fat people aren't supposed to be eating candy bars," she said. "So how can I have a whole drawer full of them?"

Seeing that everyone seemed to agree, Marti was very forceful in her reply, "No matter how much you weigh, no one has the right to tell you what you can, or cannot eat! Food is fuel for your body – and you have the right to eat any kind of food."

Taken aback at the strength of Marti's assertion, there was a flurry of reactions. Bobbie demurred, "I don't know that I could say that to Garth." Or to anyone else, she was thinking. But Marti was not going to back down – establishing boundaries and limits were vital to these women's success. To Bobbie, she said, "It's hard to visualize yourself saying that to him, but if the situation comes up again, now you have the choice of running away, or saying something. What's important is that you purchased what you wanted to eat, and you bought more than enough to reassure yourself that if you wanted some, it would be there. Right?"

"Yes." Bobbie replied.

"The point here is that deprivation leads to eating because we fear never having the opportunity again – which is eating unconsciously. So we're teaching ourselves that food is plentiful and that it's not going to disappear. Without the fear that it will evaporate, we don't have to eat when we aren't physically hungry." Bobbie, still thinking that over, said that she would give it a try. Then, she too, was finished.

Margaret volunteered to go next. Looking at her, Julie thought that here was a woman who'd had a wonderful life, happily married to a successful attorney for 33 years. It must have been so nice, Julie fantasized, staying home alone with the children all week, then having romantic weekends with her husband. And Margaret was always so beautifully dressed. Dreaming on, Julie thought about Margaret's love of her granddaughter. How lucky Devon was. This brought Julie's thoughts back to herself. I wish that I'd had a grandmother like Margaret, she thought. Maybe things would have been different for me and Eric.

Fortunately, Margaret sidetracked Julie's darkening thoughts by saying, "This was an interesting week. I went ahead and bought three containers of ice cream. But it was all gone in four days. That left me with two days that I had to go without." Together, Kate and Emily asked, "Why didn't you buy more?" Their suggestion startled Margaret. "It's so embarrassing," she said. "I hate going through the checkout counter even when I'm buying healthy things. Because of my size, when I buy things like ice cream, people look at me funny. The truth is," she said, her face saddening, "I'm always afraid that someone will actually say something to me. You know, something like, 'No wonder you're so fat!' So that's why I didn't buy any more."

Listening and watching, Marti knew that Margaret had not gotten the message. So she said, "It's nobody's business what you buy! It's your body and no one has any right to comment on it, or on the food that you buy or eat!" This time, the others supported Marti's statement.

"So nobody has a right to say anything to you or any of us," echoed Kate, loving the sound of what she was saying.

Margaret, wanting to feel as strongly as they appeared to feel, went on with the rest of her week. Her problem, she said, was that she almost never cooked for herself. "I don't feel that it's worth it to cook just for myself," she said. Emily wanted to know what she ate, then, and Margaret replied that sometimes she popped a frozen dinner into the microwave or opened a can of something. But usually, she snacked off and on all day. Responding to that, Marti said, "It's so sad that you would feel that you aren't worth the effort." That was the last thing Margaret expected. And it hit her. Hard! Then, somewhere inside, she felt the oddest thing. It was as if, in mentioning sadness, Marti had opened a door into the deepest part of her. With that door ajar, Margaret had an unexpected view of everything that was inside. She could feel all sorts of emotions swirling around. But the only one she could attach a word to was sorrow, and that was because it was always with her. Suddenly reluctant to look any closer, she couldn't speak. But Julie could.

Seeing the torment being endured by the heroine of her imagination, Julie thought how unfair it was that this wonderful woman didn't understand how important she was. So she said, "You really are worth the time and trouble." Margaret nodded, still not wanting to speak. But she was relieved, knowing that the girl was drawing attention away from her and onto herself.

Hesitantly, Julie was saying, "I did everything I thought I was supposed to. I bought enough food and had it at home and work, but I feel like I lost control one day." Sorry that she'd begun, Julie stopped here. But everyone looked at her so encouragingly, that she resumed. "Normally, I go to one school or another. But that morning, I had to visit several sites and I didn't get finished when I thought. By the time I got back to the office it was three o'clock and I'd missed lunch." Emily couldn't imagine missing lunch and she said, "I would have been starved!"

"I was," Julie said. Her voice fell away. Looking at Marti for reassurance, she continued. "This is really embarrassing, but by the time I got back I was so hungry that I…." Halting, again, she forced herself to say, "that I started eating the minute I got inside the lunchroom door." Plunging on now, she said, "I was so glad to see that there were some donuts left that I ate two before I got to my sandwich and pear." Having said all that, she stopped, waiting for judgment. But all Marti said was, "Did you enjoy everything?"

Had she? Julie wondered. Then, wanting to be as honest as possible, she said, "The donuts were stale. And I don't even remember what kind of sandwich I'd brought, or whether my pear was ripe or not." All that was true. What she did remember, however, is that the food hadn't been enough to erase the hunger pangs either. So she'd bought a candy bar from the vending machine and ate it, too.

Marti's next question took her back to early morning. "When did you have breakfast?"

"6:30 that morning."

"So there you were, without food for eight and a half hours. How do you think anyone's body would feel after not being fed that long?"

"I guess," Julie said, "my body would be famished."

"And when your body is famished, you start eating whatever is in sight!" Marti pointed out.

Having identified what had happened, Marti wanted to explain it further. "It's so important that we look at our day and plan ahead so that we know that, no matter where we are, we will have enough food. One way to do that is to carry a snack in your purse. That way, you'll always have something to take care of your physical hunger and will prevent you from feeling starved by the time you have a chance to eat a meal." Julie had never thought of doing that. "I always pack snacks and stuff for the kids, but never considered doing it for myself."

"Is that what you do?" Julie asked.

"Yup," Marti replied. "In my office, I always have my favorite cup-of-soup and crackers in case I can't leave for lunch. In my purse, I carry a granola bar or hard candies." Julie couldn't help but stifle a giggle at a picture of her favorite food – mashed potatoes. She could see them everywhere – in her purse, her car, her desk, in the mailbox. It struck her that this was the first time in nearly a year that she'd felt like really laughing. But Marti was moving on.

"Your body only knows that food is plentiful if you make sure that food is available whenever it needs it. When you wait until you're famished to begin eating, you can't enjoy the food, and you have no idea when you're full. So eating becomes an out-of-control, unsatisfying experience." Surprised at being praised for her efforts even when she wasn't doing a perfect job, Julie smiled. "Thank you," she said, "I'm finished."

Nodding, Marti went over to a stack of notebooks on a table, saying, "This week, we want you to eat at four of your favorite places. You might want to go to an old favorite or new restaurant. You might choose a favorite meal at home, fast-food, or go to a party. While you are there, we want you to envision yourself as an investigator. Notice how your body reacts to everything from the noise level to the spaces between tables. What you want to know, is why your body prefers this restaurant over all others. Is it the food? The lighting? Decor, or type of people who frequent the place, or maybe the service? I'll give you an example from one of our previous groups to help you get the idea."

Marti went on to tell about a woman who chose her favorite fast-food restaurant. "While there, she ordered her food, ate it, and left. At the time, she thought everything had been wonderful. Later, however, when she was doing her journal, she realized that there were a few things she hadn't liked: the way the restaurant smelled was one. Talking about this in group, she remembered feeling hurried and suddenly understood that she'd felt that way because everyone else seemed in such a rush. Thinking back, she wondered if she'd eaten too much because half an hour after eating, her body didn't feel as energetic as she would have liked. So, her investigator concluded that eating too much, too fast, equaled less enjoyment. That didn't mean that fast food was bad for her, but that eating fast food too fast had an adverse affect on her body. As for the odor, she decided that it had affected her enjoyment of the meal. From then on, she would order take-out at that particular chain and eat on the patio."

Looking around the table, Marti saw that there were mixed feelings about this. There was the old fear of losing control, of course. But Marti kept on going. "No matter what kind of restaurant you choose, be sure to ask your body exactly what it wants before, during, and after you've eaten. Be particularly aware of the tastes, textures, smells, and flavors of everything you eat," Marti said. "Recognize how your body responds to these differences because the only way any of us learns these things is by testing and asking ourselves questions. If the food didn't meet your standards, or doesn't satisfy you, you don't have to finish eating it. Remember, you deserve only the best and trying to satisfy yourself with anything less won't work."

Emily looked a little shocked. Wasn't that wasting food? But Marti was already explaining. "Up until now, you've been gaining weight on food that you probably didn't like." Well, now, Bobbie thought. That was certainly true.

Then Marti brought up something that they all did. "I know that many of you like eating in your car. This week, however, that doesn't count as one of the four experiences. We want you to go inside and enjoy the entire restaurant experience." None of this pleased Bobbie. In the first place, she didn't have the time. And, the thought of not knowing what full felt like and being in four of her favorite food places threatened her sense of control. "I'm afraid to enjoy what I eat," she said. "Maybe I won't be able to stop."

"You didn't lose control when you had enough candy bars," Marti observed.

"Maybe," Bobbie countered, "that's because I know that Garth knows about them." Marti nodded. "It is very hard to trust your body to tell you when it's full so that you can stop eating," she said.

"It's impossible!" Bobbie said, emphatically.

"I have a suggestion," Marti said. "Say you want a sandwich. As you're eating it, pause every once in a while, put your hand on your stomach, and ask your body if it's still hungry. Would it prefer something different? Would it like more salt, or ketchup? Does the food in front of you need to be changed to make it the best?"

"This is going to be really difficult to do," Bobbie replied.

"I know. It's hard to be so conscious. As the investigator, you will be making observations and collecting information that will help you determine what things influence TEAM eating, and what things enhance your enjoyment of the meal. So, as you select your four favorite places, be sure to eat only your favorite foods." Then it was time to go.

The women were unusually quiet as they left the office. Some were thinking about their favorite places to eat. Others were thinking about the food they would order. Each found it unbelievable that a weight-loss program was encouraging them to eat good, mouth-watering, delicious, regular food. It was while thinking that, that panic took over. Would they finally lose control – as they'd always feared?

CHAPTER FOUR

Do You Mean I Have a Choice?

Week Eight: Customizing Food to Lose Weight

BOBBIE BOONE STARED at the red light, unwilling to accept the 45 seconds it was going to take for it to change. As usual, she was running late. Under her breath, she muttered, "Change to green, change to green!" At the same time, her brain was busily scolding, when will you ever learn?

Like every other day, Bobbie had too much to do, with too little time. Busy with interns, patients, and meetings, she tried to steal a few minutes before leaving the hospital to write in her journal. Now, here she was, stuck in traffic, with a half-finished journal beside her! Aw, the heck with it, she told herself. She'd think about something else – like finally completing the restaurant assignment that had been due weeks before. It was a mixed experience, at best, because it had delivered little of the enjoyment she'd anticipated. Still, she had to admit that Marti was right about one thing: by being an observer of your own personal behavior, you noticed a lot of things that might have ordinarily been overlooked or disregarded. The light finally changed, calling Bobbie's attention back to the present, and to an awareness of how much time was left for her to reach Marti's office.

Already there, Kate had arrived early on purpose. She needed a few minutes to herself so she could think. About Ed, of course! Wondering where he was had been driving her crazy for a week. If he was injured, or dead, she would have been notified, so she figured he was choosing to stay away. That meant that he had left her. How could he leave the responsibility of running the business entirely up to her? That though brought up the question – what would she tell others if something critical came up? Alarmed just thinking about it, Kate wondered if Ed was gone for good. If so, what did that mean? Should she call the kids? How long could she continue acting as if he was coming back? What would she do about the house... their bills... the business? Her anxiety rising, Kate wondered if it was too early to get an attorney. And who would she get? The only ones she knew had been hired by Ed. When should she begin to take some sort of action? Tortured with all this uncertainty, Kate was almost relieved to have Emily come through the door. And when Emily said, "Boy, am I glad to see you," it made Kate feel better to have someone pleased to see her.

Forcing her problems away, Kate turned all of her attention to Emily. Almost desperately, she asked a barrage of questions, going from "How are you?" and ending with, "Did you get your daughter's dress finished?" By the time Margaret and Julie arrived a few minutes later, Kate was sufficiently distracted to put her personal worries aside.

From the minute they had locked their cars and joined steps, Margaret and Julie had been chatting away like old friends. Julie was feeling more and more comfortable with them. Julie started out by asking about Margaret's granddaughter. Then she told Margaret about her kids, too. But she didn't tell her everything. When they entered the waiting room, Julie included Kate and Emily in the conversation, too. It was this spirited exchange that greeted Bobbie when she arrived. As Marti opened the inner door a few seconds later, she was pleased to see that everyone was there right on time.

As she often did, Emily was the one to start. About her week, she said, "Everyone had the flu, so the clinic was a madhouse. But I really want to talk about what happened yesterday." As everyone settled in, she went on to say that, around 10:00, she'd driven to the bank to make a deposit. "As I was going along," she said, "I heard a radio commercial for the new 'light' menu at a Mexican drive-through chain. It suddenly occurred to me that I was probably not going to be able to get away for lunch because we were so swamped. So," she said, "I decided to eat right then and there."

As Emily was describing what had happened, the little girl inside of her started screaming to be heard. She wanted to tell them that she was afraid to go without. The little girl wanted everyone to understand that if she had to sit with that empty feeling, she'd shrivel up. If she didn't get food right away, she'd surely die! But Emily could not hear her; all she knew was that she suddenly felt like crying.

"I didn't have time to go inside the restaurant," Emily was saying, "So I ordered two tacos at the drive-through." Kate, who'd seen the commercials on television asked, "Were they any good?"

"They were all right," Emily said. "But I knew even before I ordered that I wasn't really hungry. I ate them anyway, because I knew that it would be my last chance."

Impressed with the insight Emily was gaining, Marti commented, "Recognizing that you ate when you weren't physically hungry is really good, Emily. Every one of us can relate to eating to stave off hunger later on. How did you feel when you realized there wasn't going to be time to eat lunch?" This wasn't something Emily needed to think over. "Scared!" she replied. Hearing this, Bobbie thought how often she did the same thing. Whenever everything got busy in ER, she feared that she wouldn't have time to eat later on. It rather flew in the face of Camilla's favorite homily, which was that being busy kept one's mind off hunger.

At the same time, Marti was thinking that Emily had never felt that it was all right for her to demand time to take care of her personal needs – especially hunger. Yet she was consciously anxious about there not being food when she got ready to eat. Deciding that Emily would be best helped by focusing on the feelings, Marti replied, "It is scary thinking you will have to go without food – that you will be stuck with that hungry, starving feeling inside. So, Emily, did eating those tacos help take care of the problem?"

The others waited for Emily's answer. It took a few minutes, then she said, "I remember that I felt uncomfortable for the rest of the morning; I felt really full." Then something else came back to her. "You know, by the time I got back to the office, I'd lost my usual morning energy." Seeing the others nodding, she knew that it had happened to them, too. Wanting to tie this together, Marti said, "It sounds like you ate ahead of time because you were afraid you might be hungry later. And it worked: you didn't feel hungry later. In fact, you felt too full and, you had no energy when you needed it most! So, was it worth it?"

"No, I didn't feel very good for the rest of the day," Emily replied.

Knowing that this could be either a physical or emotional reaction, Marti said, "The problem with trying to eat in advance is that when lunchtime comes you might still feel deprived because you didn't get to take a break. You might not be physically hungry, but there are other hungers that need to be addressed. When work gets so demanding that you don't have a chance to care for those other hungers, deprivation can become a real issue. Not having enough of anything can be difficult to deal with."

From everyone's response, Marti could see that this situation was a familiar one. So she decided to discuss it more fully. "We are tempted to eat every hour of the day. When Emily heard that commercial and knew she might not have time to eat later on, eating seemed like a good idea. But, it wasn't her body telling her that. It was an outside influence, reminding her she wouldn't have time to eat later on. What happened next was that she ate inaccurately for her body because she was unconsciously responding to Time and Emotion."

Looking around, Marti saw that her words had struck a chord. "Just thinking about being without and being hungry can dredge up old memories of deprivation at other times when we felt helpless to provide for ourselves. That's when your little girl can feel so desperate that she grabs whatever food is at hand. The sad thing is that this desperation may have nothing to do with physical hunger!" Checking around the table to make sure that everyone was following, Marti suggested, "The next time this happens, it will be important to reassure your little girl that the awful feelings and fears will go away. Tell her that there is plenty of food available to you any time you need it. Be sure to remind her that not being able to eat is only temporary because you will take steps to provide for the real hungers."

"Remember," Marti went on, "whenever your little girl panics, the adult part of you needs to promise her that you won't ever forget her, much less deprive her of what she needs. Tell her that she can always trust you to set aside a few minutes for a snack when there isn't time for a meal. And then remember to follow through and feed her. Never lie to your little girl!" Seeing that Bobbie and Kate appeared uncomfortable with what she just said, Marti rephrased it. "In other words, in a situation like this, you need to be able to take a deep breath and say to yourself that it's going to be okay, feelings are just feelings and they will pass, you can trust yourself to find ways and make time to satisfy your hungers whenever you need to satisfy them and even if you can't have everything you want right away, it doesn't mean that ultimately you won't get exactly what you want. You might have to compromise by giving yourself some time." When Bobbie and Kate relaxed, Marti knew that she had succeeded in making sense to them.

Emily said that she would remember this. Continuing with her week, she said, "There's something else that I need to talk about. The minute I get home after work, I get dinner started. But even when I've had lunch, I still find myself nibbling and sampling what I'm cooking." Her distress growing, she said, "Back when I was doing it unconsciously, I was eating low-calorie food for dinner. Now, with all this snacking and sampling – and eating regular food, too – I've gained five pounds since I started the program."

Not surprised, Marti said, "I know that it's frightening to gain weight," she said. "But it's not bad to gain at this point because it's part of learning how to understand what your body is trying to tell you. In time," she promised, "as you use our tools more accurately, the weight will come off!" Wanting to believe her, Emily decided that she better tell something that was even more difficult to reveal.

Averting her eyes so that she wasn't looking at anyone, Emily confessed, "I try not to snack in the evening. Then sometimes around two in the morning, I find myself heading straight for the kitchen." Hearing herself say that out loud made Emily feel even worse. Her voice rising, she wailed, "So I'm not just double-eating, I'm triple-eating!" She waited to hear what the others would say. But only Marti spoke. "Are you eating what you really want for dinner?" she asked.

To Emily, the question seemed to be unrelated to her problem. Still, she answered Marti's question as directly as she could. "I'm eating more healthfully," she said. "Most nights I have a really big salad; sometimes with canned tuna, or chicken." There, she thought, I hope that's the right answer. It must not have been because Marti asked another question. "But," she said, "was that what you really wanted?" Emily had to admit that it was not. "If I ate what I wanted, it would be the pork chops and roasts and scalloped potatoes I fix for everyone else." Marti was not going to let this go by and asked, "So why don't you eat that?"

Emily was astonished. "If I sat down and ate what my family eats, they'd go into shock," she said. "They'd stare at every bite I took." Kate had been listening to all this in disbelief. "Why wouldn't your family want you to eat what you cook for them?" she asked. "Because," Emily replied, "they think that someone my size shouldn't eat anything but diet food and salads!"

Sirens went off in Marti's head. Emily was transferring to her husband and children the restrictions placed on her by her parents. So Marti rephrased what Emily had said. "You are saying that you believe that no one will allow you to eat regular food, not even you. Believing that makes it difficult to convince yourself that you can have any food that you want because you see regular food as bad for you. But, Emily, food is just food!" With everything in the open, now, Emily wasn't buying that simple an answer. Speaking from her heart, she said, "If I eat what other people eat, I'll gain more weight."

All around the table, the reaction was the same. "You've got to be kidding," Kate exploded. Margaret and Julie were equally outraged. "You have every right to eat what you want," Margaret said. But Bobbie, who also feared what others might think, was relieved that neither Garth or her mother was around enough to monitor her. Her mother tried, but it didn't work, and when Garth was home, he did all the cooking and he expected her to eat everything he cooked. So she did. Now, she listened as Margaret elaborated, "A person's size has nothing to do with eating the foods they like," she said. Hearing her, Marti smiled; they were using what they were learning. Margaret went on. "Emily," she said, "you deserve to eat whatever you want!" Julie got involved, too, although with a question. "Don't you get sick and tired of nothing but salads?" she asked.

All eyes turned to Emily to see her chin begin to wobble. Everyone stopped talking. Gracefully, Marti intervened. "Could there be any connection between nibbling while you're fixing dinner, eating what you don't want for dinner, and getting up in the middle of the night to snack?" For the life of her, Emily couldn't see one. Marti waited, giving her time to think. Finally, Emily said, "There might be." Then she paused, reconsidering what had always been, to her, a way of life. "Sneaking food," she explained, "is the only thing that ever worked for me. There was no other way of getting what I wanted." She stopped again. What she'd said was true.

Marti anticipated this. And she knew the importance of having Emily examine even closer what had just been uncovered. So she said, "As you were speaking, I could see a little girl checking around to make sure no one was looking so that she could snatch what she wanted to eat. I saw her hiding in order to eat what she'd taken, and eating it so fast that she didn't have a chance to enjoy it. But speed was important because she never knew when she'd get the chance again."

Emily was astounded. How did Marti know? It was as if she'd been an invisible companion on those forays for food. Astonishment merged with another feeling – one Emily could not identify. But, overwhelmed by it, she began to cry. Had her eyes been clear, and had she looked around, she would have seen that everyone else was teary-eyed, too. But Marti, seeing that Emily had reached a moment of truth, was prepared to move her even further along for, in understanding, comes resolution.

"It's understandable that your little girl is tempted to sneak a bit of this or that when she's around regular food. And your background explains why, after everyone is asleep, she feels the need to get more. All along, regular food was what she really wanted! But," Marti continued, "sneaking bits and pieces keeps her on the outside, keeps her from belonging, robs her of the chance to enjoy anything." Emily, tears still streaming down her face, cried, "It's true. But I don't know what else to do." Fortunately, Marti had a suggestion.

"There's a big difference between your childhood and today. When you were a child, there was no one around to help you. It is very different now because you have an adult in you who can help take care of your feelings, wants, needs, and wishes. So working with the child, the adult can see the choices available in every situation."

"Choices?" Emily repeated.

"Exactly," Marti replied. "Your adult can choose to eat what your body really wants. She can choose to eat it along with everybody else. Or, she can choose to continue sneaking it, eat it alone, and never enjoy a single mouthful! She can choose to belong, or continue to be separate and alone."

Emily thought this over carefully. All of it was beginning to make sense, and she could see that it may already be happening. Excited at the possibility, she wanted to tell everyone. "I know my time is almost up, but I've got to tell you one last thing. Last week I had another chance at the restaurant assignment, and it turned out differently because I did things differently." Emily went on to explain that her office staff had gone for lunch at the same soup and salad place she'd gone to before. The first time, she'd selected only those items she thought she should eat, not what she really wanted. "But, this time," she said, "I took only what really looked good to me. I was a little embarrassed with what I'd chosen, but all the while," she said, "I kept telling myself that this was an experiment. I was an investigator who was responsible for noticing everything. And you know what?" she asked, by now dry-eyed and nearly able to smile, "No one even noticed what I was eating. Can you believe that? Or, if they did, they didn't say anything."

Had this not been such a revelation for Emily, her amazement would have been funny. "And, I had a really good time," she went on, "and I didn't feel like I was out of control."

"This is good," Marti said. "What was it like to eat exactly what you wanted?"

"I took my time and enjoyed every bite," said Emily. "I didn't finish everything, which is kind of strange because I've always felt driven to clean my plate."

"So, when you ate what you really wanted, you felt more satisfied and ate less than you normally do?" Emily nodded and Marti asked, "How did your body feel after the meal?"

"Well," Emily said, all signs of earlier distress gone, "I didn't have that heavy I-want-to-take- a-nap feeling. And I didn't get hungry in the afternoon, either."

"So choosing to eat what you really wanted alongside your colleagues did several things: It allowed you to enjoy the food. You felt part of the group. You didn't get that gnawing, hungry feeling afterward, so you didn't need to nibble and snack later." Emily smiled. "That's true," she said. But Marti wasn't finished.

"In addition, you enjoyed the experience and you found that you ate less than you expected to." Emily sighed and relaxed back into her chair. "Right again!" she said. Smiling, too, Marti said, "The best part about this, Emily, is that when you begin eating for your body at every meal, your extra weight will start coming off." Feeling more confident than she had for a long time, Emily wanted to shout that she could – she would – do it. But, as much as she wanted to, could she? Stricken with sudden doubt, Emily was glad that her time was over. Much to her relief, Emily heard Bobbie say, "I'll go next."

"I finally got time to complete the restaurant assignment," she said, in a tone that told everyone that she was both apologizing for not having done it on time, but pleased with herself for doing it at all. "It didn't turn out to be what I expected, but I learned a lot," she said. "I have always wanted to try the curry buffet at a East Indian restaurant, but I never made a reservation because I wasn't sure that I could keep it. One night last week, I had gotten out of work on time and Garth was out of town. I decided to chance there being room without a reservation and went to the restaurant." "What was it like?" Kate wanted to know. Bobbie enjoyed describing what she'd seen. "It was right out of the Arabian Nights," she said. "With cane furniture, tall palms, feathered fans overhead, and waiters in turbans."

Warming up to her subject, Bobbie went on. "The buffet tables were beautifully laid out with white damask cloths and at least a dozen silver chafing dishes full of the most delicious-smelling meats, sauces, and side dishes that you can imagine. There were bowls filled with different kinds of chutneys and chopped herbs too many to name. And everything smelled so good that my mouth watered. I stood there waiting to be seated, wondering where I was going to start."

"Sounds exotic," observed Margaret, filing the information away for future use; maybe she could get Bob to go there sometime. "It was," Bobbie admitted, "and it was exciting to try something new." Then she told them about being seated in the dining room. She'd been glad, she said, that the chairs were so roomy. She had barely sat down when a waiter appeared with the menu. "But I didn't need it," Bobbie said, "because I was going to help myself at the buffet. First, I sat there being an investigator. I asked myself all sorts of questions, but I found it difficult to decide whether my body was hungry, or was I responding to the looks and smells of everything." Kate grinned, thinking that for someone who was always rushed, Bobbie sure noticed a lot of details.

Bobbie went on to describe how it felt being in the buffet line. "I stood there for a minute, just inhaling everything," she said. "Then I started down the line, taking whatever caught my fancy. Halfway through, I realized that my plate had run out of room. Actually, I'd heaped so much on it that it formed a rather embarrassing mound. And that made me aware of the other people in line – what must they be thinking? So I went back to my table to enjoy what I had, planning to go back for a new plate when I'd finished the first. Then I found that I didn't like a lot of what I'd chosen. I finished what I liked and signaled for the waiter to come and take my plate away."

"Good for you," Emily said.

Pleased at her approval, Bobbie smiled at Emily. Then, sobering, she said, "I wanted to go right back to the buffet and get the rest of the things, but I'd been there just a few minutes before and thought my being there again so soon would look funny. Before I could do anything, the waiter was looking at my nearly full plate, and he kept asking me something. Only I couldn't understand him, so I said, 'Excuse me?' He gave me a frustrated look, repeating himself, a little slower and louder, this time: 'Didn't you like it?' he shouted." Saying that, Bobbie heard a gasp from the Group. Looking around, she saw that everyone understood what had gone on, for they had long feared the same type of thing happening to them. Relieved, Bobbie said, "I was mortified. Everyone heard him! So, speaking as softly as I could, I told him that I wanted to try some of the other things. He took the plate away, but I know that he thought I was crazy. And I sat there for a few minutes, not knowing what to do. Should I leave? Or, should I go back to the buffet and pick up where I left off – except that for sure everybody would be watching now." For the Group, it was hard to wait for Bobbie's decision. Marti asked first. "What did you choose to do?"

"I asked myself if I was still hungry," Bobbie said. "And myself said yes – and there were things on that buffet that I hadn't tasted yet. So I got up, telling myself as I did that I wasn't going to let anyone tell me what to do, think, or say." Hearing her determination, it occurred to Marti that what Bobbie was saying might go beyond the waiter and the other patrons. It might even go beyond food. I wonder, Marti thought, who else in Bobbie's life tries to control her? Bobbie was going on, grinning now. "Everything I took the second time around was wonderful," she said. "Not too hot and not too bland. But no matter how good it tasted, I couldn't eat it all."

Before Marti had a chance to inquire, Emily asked, "Did the waiter say anything to you about the leftovers this time?"

"Not a word!" Bobbie replied, "He looked at me funny, but I just smiled, thanked him, and left feeling really good about everything."

Thinking that it couldn't get much better than that, Marti said, "Good for you, Bobbie, for not letting anyone intimidate you into leaving, or eating more than you really wanted. So, what was your overall impression of that experience?" Growing serious, Bobbie said, "What I enjoyed most was eating somewhere calm and peaceful – and pretty. It was a far cry from trying to eat in ER, where it's noisy, chaotic, and institutional. I ate everything I wanted and it was the right amount because I felt good when I left. Often, I feel overly full, and that's probably why I didn't get sick this time, either. While I love spicy foods, they usually don't agree with me. Now, I'm thinking that I probably ate too much before. And maybe too fast."

Marti was gladdened by Bobbie's self-analysis and conclusions. "Remaining conscious appears to have made a big difference in the way you eat," she said. This, and the Group's obvious admiration, filled Bobbie with a sense of accomplishment. And then, peeking at her watch, she saw that she had enough time to talk about something that was really bothering her. "Last night, when I got home from work, I could hear the TV in the den and knew that Garth was home." This was new – while Bobbie had always shared her frustrations with her job, she'd never talked about Garth before. Well, each thought, was Bobbie finally trusting them?

"Standing in the kitchen," Bobbie was saying, "I got a whiff of the dinner he was fixing. It smelled wonderful. Then I noticed that he'd put my mail on the counter. So, before letting him know I was home, I started leafing through the envelopes. Most were bills – one from Nordstrom's." Here in her story, Bobbie divulged a secret. "I've had an account there forever, but I don't buy much at their main store. I make do with what's on sale at their discount showroom." Marti wondered why Bobbie felt the need to explain that. What else, mused Marti, is Bobbie trying to tell us?

Moving along, Bobbie said, "So you can imagine how stunned I was to find a whole list of charges listed that amounted to $950!" Her shock was immediately magnified by the surprise on everyone else's face. That helped Bobbie continue. "Right away," she said, "I checked to see what the items were. There was a $600 man's suit, two shirts and ties, and a half dozen socks. I almost had a stroke, until it occurred to me that I'd picked up Garth's bill by mistake. But when I went to put it back in the envelope, I saw my name and account number at the top." Around the table, no one moved; what, three of them were wondering, would they do in a situation like this? "Except," Bobbie went on, "it didn't make sense because Garth has his own Nordstrom's account. And my card was in my drawer. At least, I thought it was. I just stood there for a few minutes," she said, "so upset that I couldn't think straight." Kate, who'd more than once been similarly surprised, thought that she knew what that felt like!

"Well," Bobbie continued, "I took a couple of deep breaths and put the bills back on the counter. Then I went into the den where Garth was having his martini and watching the news. The minute he saw me, he smiled really wide and said, 'Hi, Bobbsie.' He was so happy to see me that I didn't have the heart to bring up the charges." Then, wanting them to understand why she couldn't, Bobbie said, "We have so little time together that I didn't want to upset him. And he was so eager to pour me a glass of wine and ask me all the right questions about my day. And then the timer went off and he went into the kitchen for dinner. Seeing him fussing around in there, I knew that I had a good ten minutes alone. I sat there, feeling bad because I was going to have to ruin everything by bringing up those charges. I was really torn, you know? On the one hand, it was embarrassing to have to discuss this at all – I've always hated talking about money. But then, why should I get stuck with his bill? He should have asked me first. Then I got scared – what if he can't pay me back? The thought of this expense on top of everything else made my hands sweat. I didn't know how I'd do it; there isn't much left at the end of the month. So, I was trying to figure this out when he called me to the table.

"Garth," Bobbie explained, "is truly a gourmet cook. So dinner was a copy of a meal he'd had at a restaurant the week before. The problem is, he goes to those nouvelle cuisine places that serve really beautiful – but small – portions. Mind you, I hadn't eaten since breakfast, and that was only a cinnamon roll, and I'm looking at three baby carrots placed like arrows around a filet mignon that's about the size of a silver dollar. There was a tablespoon of sauce over it, and half a baked acorn squash with some grilled herbs to one side. And there Garth was, waiting for applause. Since I didn't want to hurt his feelings, I couldn't say 'Is that all there is?' So, I told him it was wonderful, sat down, and polished off every single bite – even the squash, which I hate. But it wasn't nearly enough because I was still hungry. Dessert would have helped, but Garth never thinks of that because he doesn't like sweets. But before the panic set in, I reminded myself that I could have a candy bar from my supply. Then I knew that it was time to talk to him about the bill." Sitting there, Margaret couldn't help but wonder why Bobbie didn't have any money at the end of the month. Because Garth had taken Bobbie's credit card without permission, Kate wanted to warn Bobbie; once you've started underwriting a man, it's impossible to stop. The guy's a leech, she wanted to say, get rid of him!

At the same time, Emily said to herself, I sure know what it feels like to be finished with a meal and still be hungry. For Julie, however, the entire subject revolved around Bobbie's ability to discuss money with Garth. In their house, Tom handled everything. Not that she wanted to, Julie thought; the last thing she wanted to worry about was paying bills.

Unaware of all this conjecture, Bobbie said, "I'm sitting there, knowing this is my only chance because he's going back on the road again and I won't have enough money to pay the bill myself. I don't want my credit to be ruined. So, I took a deep breath and said, 'I got the Nordstrom's bill today, and there are charges on it that I didn't make. Do you know anything about it?' And he looked at me with those big, blue eyes, and said, 'Oh Bobbsie, darling, I meant to tell you about that.' It turns out that he used my account because he had reached the limit on his own. I've got to tell you," she said, relief written all over her face, "I couldn't believe it; first that he'd owned up to it, and second that he wasn't the least bit angry that I wanted to talk about it!" Then, sensing that everyone was waiting for her to say more, she explained further. "He told me that he never meant to worry me, and that he'd already planned to make the monthly payments. Then we watched TV together. But," she had to admit, "I was still hungry so, before I went to bed, I had a candy bar."

All the time Bobbie was talking, she was thinking that maybe she'd been wrong to mention being financially strapped. Should she, if they asked, tell them that – in addition to her mortgage and college loans – she was paying for Garth's Mercedes? Even her mother didn't know that! The good news was that her own car was paid for, and Garth picked up the tab for his own gas and maintenance. Ruminating about this, Bobbie was called back to the present by Marti, who was complimenting her.

"You did the right thing, Bobbie," Marti said. "It's important to have boundaries and limits because they define who we are, as well as what we expect from others. When anyone oversteps our limits, it's important to speak to them about it. When it's someone we love it's even more important to talk about it to protect the relationship. We do it to show that we care." This was good news to Bobbie, for it had become important to her to have the support of Marti and the others. But, suddenly she was fatigued. Giving everyone a small smile, she said "Thank you. And that's it for me." Kate said she'd be next.

It had been a pretty good week, Kate thought to herself. Except for Ed, but she wasn't going to mention any of that! Instead, she talked about the week's assignment. For instance, she'd noticed that a lot of the decisions she made about food were based upon outside sources like aromas coming from restaurants and shops, or just hearing about a restaurant or food item. Even as she was saying this, though, a part of her was longing to spill the beans on Ed. But even though she'd been pretty outspoken about him before, it took more courage than she had at the moment to say out loud that he'd left her. So she continued with the assignment.

"I've stopped eating in my car," she claimed. "It wasn't easy because I've always liked the privacy of it. But, this past week I ended up spilling my drink all over." Unexpectedly, she was angry. Just as angry as she'd been when it happened. "There just isn't enough room in cars to spread out and eat comfortably," she said. "So, now I either have to go inside, take it back to the office, or bring it home to eat." Not surprisingly, Marti said, "You can still eat in the car if you want to!" Taken aback, Kate replied, "I could, but I won't." There was a pause, and then she confessed, "I hate the smell of old fast food in my car!" Everyone agreed except Bobbie, who'd never thought about it before. Did her car reek?

Laughing, Marti said, "That's wonderful. It sounds like you've made a decision to enjoy your meals instead of eating them in a cramped, little space." It felt good to be acknowledged, Kate thought. And then she couldn't hold back any longer. She could feel the support from everyone and decided to tell them about Ed's disappearance. Hearing of it, they all worried about her first. Then, they were furious with him. "How could he do that to you?" demanded Margaret, thinking that Kate deserved more. Someone supportive, like Bob, Margaret thought. Emily was equally livid. Her own husband, Dave, was not perfect by any stretch of the imagination, but he wouldn't just up and leave. Julie felt a wave of intense feeling. She didn't like it – divorce, or even the hint of divorce, always sent her into a panic. To protect herself from that sort of reality, her mind retreated back to the novel she'd started reading the night before. Unaware of the conversation that followed, she was startled back into the moment when Marti asked, "With Ed gone, have you found yourself eating any differently?"

Slowly, Kate swung around to face Marti, saying, "Well, I haven't binged." Only then did she realize that this was so. "With him not being around, it didn't seem to make much sense to cook. So I ate what I wanted, and when I wanted it. One night, a friend from our old neighborhood called and asked us over for barbecue. I told her that Ed was out of town, but I'd come alone if that was all right. And you know what? We had a better time without him." Kate gave one of her short, brusk laughs as she said this. While everyone believed that was true, they knew that Kate didn't really think it was funny. Going on, Kate said, "I still snacked in front of TV after dinner, but I ate less than usual, and not as often. The thing that worries me," she said, "is that I don't know if all that will change if and when he comes back."

Proud of Kate for risking a look at her relationship with Ed, Marti knew it was time to find out how that related to food. "Do you think there might be a connection between your food and your husband?" she asked.

"I was afraid you'd ask that," Kate said. This time, she didn't laugh. When she spoke again, her voice no longer carried its usual brittleness. Now, everyone could see what lay behind the veneer that had protected her for so long. Pain accompanying every word, Kate said, "I'm going to have to start thinking about that, aren't I?" Wanting to let Kate know how much she cared about her, Margaret said, "If Bob treated me the way your husband treats you, I don't know what I'd do."

"I don't either," Emily breathed. And, for the briefest of moments, Kate allowed herself to ask herself why she was so willing to tolerate Ed's behavior, either. But what she thought was, You guys don't understand how difficult this is. When you've been married as long as we have, you don't just get a divorce.

Looking at her, Marti saw tears threatening to spill over. Then Kate spoke, but her eyes were fastened on her folded hands rather than on any of them. "I'm finished now. Let someone else talk." The abruptness with which she said this told Marti that anything about Ed was a topic they'd have to enter gently. And she, Marti thought, would have to remain alert to what any such discussion might stir up in others. Then Julie volunteered to go next.

"One night last week Tom and I decided to go out again," she said. "Only this time we went without the kids. That's a big change for us. I was kind of afraid that we wouldn't have anything to talk about." Hurrying on, Julie said, "I found out that I eat differently without the children."

Margaret couldn't let that one go by. "I remember how wonderful it was to eat an occasional meal alone with my husband," she said."There's a lot to be said about eating in a calm, orderly, beautiful place, with people to wait on you." Wistfully, Emily asked, "Is there such a place?" Even as the others laughed at the poignant way she'd said this, Emily was thinking that she and Dave never went anywhere without the kids. Julie was so thrilled about Margaret identifying with her situation that she felt less nervous about sharing more of her discoveries.

"I finally realized that I don't like the food my kids and Tom want. In the restaurant, Tom ordered his usual steak and potatoes. The kids like the same foods; you know, like steak, hamburgers, macaroni and cheese, pizza, hot dogs, and fried chicken. But I like variety. I get tired of the same, old food. So it was exciting to look at the menu with all the choices. That made me aware of how boring it is to eat at home." Wanting to understand more, Marti asked, "Give us an example of a meal you had last week."

Happy to do that, Julie said, "Last night we had hamburger patties in gravy, and mashed potatoes with peas and sliced carrots. Well," she sighed, "the kids didn't like the vegetables and kept asking if they had to eat them. My son got so upset that he spilled his milk, and my daughter kept insisting that I give her ding-dongs instead. It got to the point where I couldn't stand it anymore. So I gave them their ding-dongs and sent them in to watch TV. Then – and this is what worries me – while I was clearing off the table, I ate everything they'd left on their plates! But, that's not the worst," she added, embarrassed to be telling this. "I ate all the ding-dongs that were left, too." Miserably, she hung her head, even though she'd not told them how many packages she'd eaten, or that she'd continued snacking until she'd gone to bed. But Marti wasn't interested in that. "Tell us more about what it's like for you to eat with the children," she said. Uncomfortable all of a sudden, Julie said, "Sometimes the noise they make and their constant demands are more than I can bear and I want to get away from them. But I can't blame them for doing what kids do. So I end up feeling guilty because only bad moms want to escape from their children. I'm afraid that if my kids find out that I don't want to be around them, I will have damaged them, somehow."

Wanting Julie to see that setting reasonable limits is not harmful to children, Marti said, "One of the most difficult jobs parents have is in teaching children what is expected of them. We do that by letting them know what our limits are: when we're eating at the table we do this – and we don't do that! This really helps them later on when they have to eat with others."

"Sometimes," Julie admitted, "I feel like what's the use, they don't listen to me anyway. But, lately, it just makes me mad."

"Of course," Marti agreed. "Everyone feels angry when they're being ignored." But she knew there was more to this than had been said when Julie whispered, "What do I do with this anger!" Now Kate stepped in. "Does your husband help out at dinnertime?"

For some reason, the question made Julie feel that she had to defend Tom."I don't think he knows what to do, either. So he leaves all the rule-making and discipline up to me." Marti brought that right back to the reason they were all there by asking, "Do you see any connection between eating the leftovers and ding-dongs, your choice of food for dinner, and feeling helpless and solely responsible for the control of your children's behavior?" For the first time, Julie realized there might be a link between them. That was unsettling.

The truth of the matter was that Julie had been raised to be compliant and polite and understood no other way of handling things. So she feared that if she were too demanding of anyone, they wouldn't like her, and eventually they'd leave. Even her own children. Now, feeling that she'd said more than enough, Julie deflected Marti's question by saying, "I'm going to have to look at that this next week." She was surprised when Marti didn't leave it at that. "You mentioned that you ate differently in a calm environment," she said. "That's always going to be very difficult with young children. So," she suggested, "you and your husband might want to eat at a different time." This struck Julie too close to home – she didn't want her children to have to endure what she and Eric had experienced. But, before she could object, Margaret was agreeing.

"That's what I did when my children were young," she said. "I fixed them what they wanted for dinner, then read stories to them while they ate. It was wonderful because it gave me special time with them, and time later to enjoy my own dinner." Well, now, Julie thought. Turning the kids' dinner into story time had never occurred to her. So she was more open-minded when Marti said, "It's important for kids to have some meals with the family, but it's equally important that you, Julie, eat your dinner in an atmosphere that allows you to enjoy your food. That way you can eat more consciously, which means that you won't leave the table feeling dissatisfied, or deprived, or angry."

Emily had something to say, too. "Maybe you could ask your husband for help when the kids get out of line," she said. "If he doesn't know what to do, he needs to learn because he probably doesn't like feeling helpless, either."

There were a number of surprising possibilities here, Julie thought. Maybe, if she spent more time alone with Tom, they could work together on this. Who knew, maybe they'd get some romance back in their lives. Feeling better about having brought the subject up, Julie thanked everyone, saying, "I really am going to work on this." As everyone turned to Margaret, Julie kind of drifted off, trying to remember if it was Mary Poppins, or the governess in Wuthering Heights who read to her charges during meals.

Margaret was ready to share her week with the group. After two years of withdrawing from the social scene because of her weight, she had finally agreed to attend a party at the home of one of Bob's clients. It was too bad that Julie was lost in her own thoughts because she would have loved Margaret's recounting of the event. "It was an enormous event," she said, "celebrating a multi-million dollar victory in court. Everyone in the firm, along with their spouses were invited to meet the top level people in this company. There were about 150 people for a sit-down dinner."

"How do you seat 150 people?" Emily asked, overwhelmed at the thought of planning that big an affair. "In this house, there was more than enough room – it was an enormous manor house set on acres and acres of land. Once you entered through the big, iron gates, you drove for minutes before you even saw the house. It's the kind of place you read about in Gothic novels." Slowly, Julie's attention began returning to the here and now.

"There were staff and caterers everywhere," Margaret said. "They led us through the house to a tented courtyard at the far end. Everyone was milling around outside. An orchestra was playing Cole Porter tunes, I could see inside the tent and the table settings were incredibly elaborate, so I knew that it was going to be a four- or five-course dinner. The problem was that I was hungry, I didn't know when we'd be eating, and waiters were carrying trays of champagne and the fanciest hors d'oeuvres you've ever seen. I mean," she said, "you couldn't want for anything." Foreseeing her quandary, everyone waited to see how Margaret had handled it. "I kept asking myself how many hors d'oeuvres I dared eat. And I kept wondering what Marti would suggest. So I decided to select five of the hors d'oeuvres that looked the best – and I took tiny bites instead of eating it in one gulp. And that made them last a lot longer."

"By choosing your favorites and taking smaller bites, did you find that you enjoyed them more?"

"Yes. A lot of times, I haven't even tasted appetizers. When the waiters came around with other trays, I was enjoying what I had so much that I didn't feel pressured to take more."

"So what happened with dinner?" Julie asked, living the experience along with Margaret.

"Well, it was a five-course meal, but the hostess had chosen really light-weight things, like bouillon soup, a pretty garden salad – but I didn't like the nasturtiums and other flowers because they were bitter. Then came a small plate of shellfish risotto, which was delicious and I ate it all. Although I regretted that a few minutes later when they waiters served the main course."

"What did they serve?" Kate wanted to know.

"Two large slices of four-peppered pork roast, potatoes dauphine, and miniature vegetables. It looked delicious, too." said Margaret. "I didn't know what to do. I wanted to eat every bit of it, but my dress was beginning to feel a little tight across my middle, so I knew that I was already full. Still, I couldn't leave a whole plate of untouched food, so I ate half a slice of meat, a bite of the potatoes, and I skipped the vegetables – although they looked pretty. And then, we had about an hour before dessert because there were the speeches and dancing."

"Did you dance?" asked Julie.

"Yes, Bob's quite a dancer. But what surprised me was how proud he seemed to be of me. Ever since I've gained this weight, I thought I was more an embarrassment to him than an asset. But he was eager to introduce me to everyone and happy to sit out the dancing when I got tired."

"From your description," Marti said, "it sounds like you had a wonderful time, and I am proud of you for remaining so conscious throughout the evening. Will you do anything differently the next time?"

Retracing her steps, Margaret said, "I'm glad that I didn't pig out on the hors d'oeuvres because I really enjoyed the main course. I wish I could have eaten more of it. Now that I'm thinking of it, I really could have passed up the soup and salad courses." Emily raised her hand. "How would you do that politely?" she asked.

"What I really mean is that I could have eaten less of those, or just left it," Margaret explained. "Lots of people do that. It was just hard because I didn't know what we were going to be served next."

Marti responded to Margaret's frustration. "That was a very difficult situation," she said. "Without knowing what's coming next, it is hard to know what to do. There isn't a right answer to these kinds of situations. We have to kind of play them by ear. However, it's important that you noticed that soup and salad are not going to be your favorite things at this kind of a party. What's most important is that you had a good time."

Margaret agreed. "But that's not all that happened this past week," she said. "I had Devon for a couple of days, which I just love." As she described the things they'd done, everyone smiled, thinking what a wonderful grandmother Margaret was.

Feeling the warmth of their smiles, Margaret wanted to tell them that there was a negative side of this relationship, too. Sometimes Devon's being there reminded her of what happened to her when she was five. But how could she tell anyone that when she was with Devon she found herself measuring her light-hearted zest for life with her own loss of innocence. And how do I admit, she wondered, that while I love her to pieces, sometimes I wish she wasn't there?

Thinking this, Margaret was frustrated. She really didn't want Devon to go away. If she could only find the connection between her recent weight gain and the sexual abuse, maybe things would go back to the way they were. Then, she could enjoy all of her time with Devon again. She began to wonder how long it would take to find the answer, and how long would it take to lose the weight? Aloud, she said, "I don't know about anyone else, but I haven't lost any weight, yet." It was the same for Kate, so she said, "I'm getting worried; we've been doing this for eight weeks, now!" And Emily said, "I've actually gained weight!"

"Will we ever lose this weight?" Bobbie asked.

Knowing that with dieting the old way the weight came off faster, Marti knew that she had to reassure them that permanent weight loss was different. "Finding the reasons why your weight won't come off is a process. Learning to use all the tools for eating consciously is really a big job. Because they are so new, it is going to take awhile before they become a part of you. What makes it even harder is that, at the same time, you're replacing years and years of other people's rules about food and eating with your own. Whether your weight has changed or is staying the same, it reflects your body's attempts to deal with all the changes. It takes time for your body to adjust to the fact that food is plentiful and that there isn't a famine. It also takes time to trust your body – to believe that it will tell you what it wants." Looking around, Marti saw everyone but Julie paying close attention: her attention, as it so often did, had returned to something else. This time, she was remembering a story she'd read before falling asleep last night. It was historical, of course, involving a commoner and a prince. Improbable, but romantic.

"So don't worry if you haven't lost weight yet," Marti reassured them. "It will come off as you eat more accurately to meet your body's needs. As you eat more for physical hunger, you will begin to identify the other hungers in your body and in your life. You will learn to satisfy the other hungers without using food all the time. Then you'll see your weight starting to drop away."

"And never come back?" Emily asked.

"And never come back – because, as long as you eat what you really want when you're really hungry, and continue using the tools we've learned in class, you'll be responding to your body accurately. Then your body will stay at its natural weight!" said Marti.

For some reason, what Marti said gave Margaret considerable comfort. "I really needed to hear that because I get so impatient sometimes," she said. Then, seeing by the clock that time had run out, Margaret said that she was finished, after which Marti stood to hand out the next week's assignment. As always, everyone snapped them into their notebooks as Marti said, "We've had eight weeks together and so far, you have these tools for conscious eating:

- TEAM eating

- Food Critic

- Internal cues for listening to your body

- The knowledge that food is plentiful

- Eat what you really want when you are hungry and stop when you are full.

"This next week," Marti continued, "we add one more tool: we're going to begin customizing your food so that everything you take into your body will make it feel good. That means it feels energized, alert, and light. We call this Proactive Eating. The flip side of that are foods that make you sick, give you an upset stomach, gas or diarrhea, or make you feel lethargic or tired. Those foods we need to eat at select times when it's alright to feel that way. This," she said, "is going to be different for everyone. And it will take time to find out which foods fit into which categories." Turning to the chalkboard, she wrote two headlines: "Foods That Make Me Feel Light, Alert, and Energized" and "Foods That Make Me Feel Sick." At this point, Marti sensed uneasiness in the room. Kate voiced what everyone was thinking.

"So," she said, "you're saying that if a food makes us feel sick, we shouldn't eat it!" Marti smiled, knowing all too well that this was an important test. If she agreed, they'd know their worst fears had come true – that this was just another diet. In a flash, they'd dismiss her as just one more "expert" telling them what they could and could not eat. So she answered carefully, "No, that's not what I'm saying at all. I'm saying that you have a choice. If you find yourself craving something that you know is going to make you sick, or tired, then you might not want to eat it when you want to be alert.

Instead, plan to eat it when being tired won't interfere with what you want to do!"

Looking around to see if she'd survived the inquiry, Marti was pleased to see everyone appearing relieved. Kate affirmed it by saying, "You know, I really thought this program had just taken a sudden turn and we were back to dieting. I just couldn't do it again." But Emily had a question. "How does customizing our food help us lose weight?" she asked.

Marti was quick to respond. "Customizing food helps you to fuel your body with food that will not interfere with whatever you need or want to do which will lead to a decrease in double- eating, or eating unconsciously, and that leads to weight loss. You see," she explained. "when people eat foods that make them tired or listless when they need to be alert and energetic, they may be tempted to eat a candy bar, or something, to revitalize themselves. Then they're right back to eating unconsciously – which leads to gaining weight." Smiling at them, Marti finished the evening by saying, "So, it's time to stop for tonight. Have a good week."

And week eight was over.

CHAPTER FIVE

What's Missing In My Life?

Week Ten: Identifying the Other Hungers

HE EVENING BEFORE their next meeting, Marti sat
down to review the past nine weeks. The beauty of
working with these groups, she thought, was that the
members who had been doing their homework were well
into addressing their own personal concerns. Even those not as con-
scientious about doing the work had been compelled by example to
at least face their own issues. For many, this week would mark the
point-of-no-return: never again could they go back to diets or dieting. Having become aware of the other hungers in their lives, they'd
already taken the first steps toward recognizing the real reasons
they'd gained and retained weight. Fortunately, now they were also
learning new ways, other than food, to take care of those hungers.
Ultimately, this process would lead them to permanent weight loss.

Customizing their food had been one such learning experience.
Marti was thrilled when Emily discovered how much better she felt
on the days she went without breakfast. What was better for her,
Emily found, was a mid-morning snack of toast or fruit. The hard

part had been trying to remember to take the time to eat it when everything else was demanding her attention.

Julie learned more about herself as well, finding how much better her body felt when she cut back on dairy products. For Margaret, however, answers had come more slowly. Identifying foods that made her feel sluggish had been easy, but she was still trying to isolate the foods that made her body feel good. Kate, on the other hand, continued worrying about being out of control with her late-night snacking, in spite of the fact that with Ed gone, she didn't seem to do it as much. Then there was Bobbie, who was just beginning to show signs of interest in adding variety to her old standby of fast foods. This had come into the light of day when Kate mentioned the vast range of pre-cooked foods that just needed heating in the microwave. As much as she would like to try them, Bobbie admitted that with her schedule it was going to be difficult to find the time.

Marti knew that making time for herself had always been a big problem for Bobbie. Preparing her own meals was especially difficult for her because it included setting aside time for planning, going to the store, storing, and preparing the food, far more time than it took to gulp down her usual cheeseburger while driving. But if Bobbie would try to explore different options for getting food, such as ordering from restaurants or investigating the wonderful meals now available at grocery stores, the therapist knew Bobbie would discover entirely new experiences of taste, textures, and aromas that would give her more choices to satisfy her physical hunger. Marti had confidence that Bobbie would accomplish this for herself some day soon. This brought Marti's thoughts around to tomorrow, when each of the women was to report what they'd discovered about what was missing in their lives.

This was not easy, Marti knew from experience. But when you begin identifying those things in your everyday life that aren't satisfying, you gain clues to explain why you eat when you aren't physically hungry. Hmmm, Marti mused. What reactions would she see this week when they could finally see that there was more to their weight than just food? This realization would prod them to look even deeper inside. What that frequently did, of course, was rekindle a number of feelings. For some, it might be a sense of loss. For others, there could be fear, and maybe even an overwhelming sense of responsibility. It was never easy to deal with these feelings at first. I wonder, Marti thought, how many of them ate unconsciously this week? For most, she knew, eating would be the automatic response to uncomfortable feelings.

* * * * *

After everyone had taken their usual seats, Julie surprised them all by announcing that she wanted to be first. She began with, "I did all of the exercises," she said, "except one. It had to do with talking to my extra weight – to find out why it came, and why it has stayed. Well, the only thing that came to me," she said, "was protection, but that doesn't make a whole lot of sense." Hearing this, Marti made a mental note: What threatened Julie, causing her to build a wall of protection around herself? To explore this further, she asked, "What is the danger?" Sitting there, Julie wished everyone could read her mind so she didn't have to say it. Then fear took over, and she said, "I don't know."

Marti was hoping that Julie would talk about what she was keeping locked up inside of her. But seeing the blank expression on the young woman's face, she decided not to push further. "The answer is there, inside of you," she said. "It will just take time to recognize it." Feeling a wave of relief, Julie nodded and decided to talk about something positive. "I finally did it," she said. "And it never would have happened if it hadn't been for all of you!" Then she explained. "It's been hard to admit even to myself that my kids were sometimes beyond my control." Turning directly to Marti, she explained. "A few weeks ago when we were talking about setting limits, you said that it was important for parents to be firm and consistent in their discipline. That really struck home because I wasn't consistent at all. So, I took your advice – and it really worked!" Marti smiled in acknowledgment, but Julie was already moving on, illustrating how she'd used the advice.

"You see," she explained, "when it's time for the kids to get their pajamas on they're pretty good. It's when they actually have to get into bed that they start running around the house, yelling and screaming. By the time I've gotten them quieted down and into bed, I'm so tired that I can't enjoy the rest of the evening. So this week, I laid down the law. I told them that if they didn't go to bed the minute I told them to, they would be going to bed half an hour earlier the next night."

They hadn't believed her, Julie admitted, but why should they – she'd never taken a real stand before. "But I didn't let that stop me," she told the Group. "At 8:00 the next night I turned off the TV and pointed to the hallway. And even when they whined and cried, I didn't back down or lose my temper. Instead, I reminded them very calmly about my warning the night before. 'If you don't go to bed this very instant,' I told them, 'you'll miss all of your programs tomorrow night.'" Julie reported that there were a few protests, but she'd held firm and, for the first time ever, the two were in bed on time. "The third night it wasn't much of an issue," she said, smiling. "which allowed me to have the energy to enjoy the rest of the evening. That night, I just sat and enjoyed the quiet. The next night I wandered down into the Tom's office in the basement to see what he was up to." Smilingly, she added, "Boy, was he surprised! And I think he liked having me there. He even showed me the different things he's doing on the computer." Having told them all the good stuff, Julie knew it was time to talk about what wasn't working in her life. The others, seeing her thrill of accomplishment fall away, wondered what caused her change of mood.

Soberly, Julie said, "The biggest frustration in my life is one I've had forever. It's..." She hesitated, wondering if she could go through with it. Never had she told anyone but Tom this before. Oh, she sighed, why couldn't my family be normal? But they weren't, and she needed help with the latest catastrophe. Noticing that she had everyone's attention, she felt pressure build inside. They were all waiting to hear what was bothering her. If she stopped now, she would really look stupid. So, she took a deep breath and said, "I have to tell you what happened with my mom and brother last week." The mournful way she introduced them to the others made their hearts constrict; whatever Julie was about to say was coming from the deepest, most private part of her. As interested as everyone else was, Marti's antennae flashed upward: this was the first time Julie had ever said much about her mother and brother.

Having brought the subject up, Julie was hesitant about saying more. Had she just loosened the lid on her own Pandora's box? Yet, desperate for help, she plunged on. "Last Saturday was my mom's birthday," she explained. "and against my better judgment – and warnings from my husband – I invited her and my brother to dinner." Knowing that the others would question her reluctance, Julie explained. "I really love my mom, but she has always favored my brother. In her eyes he never does anything wrong even though he is 34 years old, can't keep a job, and still lives at home. It drives me crazy that she refuses to see his problem with drugs and alcohol. It's gotten so that I hate planning anything with them because I never know what's going to happen." Again anticipating unasked questions, Julie explained. "I've tried to invite my mother to come alone," she said, "but she refuses. She's never been able to go anywhere without a man, even if it's just my brother." Seeing that everyone was trying to understand, Julie was encouraged to go on.

"I bent over backwards to make everything perfect. I got up early Saturday morning, got the kids settled in the back yard, cleaned the house, and baked her favorite cake. I set the table with our best china and silver, got flowers, and made sure that the rib roast would be ready right on time. And it worked out beautifully: at 5:30, everything was ready – down to the kids who were bathed and in their good clothes. Except that my mom and brother were nowhere to be seen. In fact, they didn't get there until 6:30. Since they hadn't called to say when they would arrive, Tom was keeping the kids quiet with videos while I was in the kitchen worrying about how to save the roast. And then in they came," Julie said, her hands illustrating how carefree their arrival had been, "with Mom making her usual grand entrance, wearing something totally inappropriate for her age just to show off her tiny, little waist. My mother always wears things that let men know that she's available. It's so embarrassing. Well, Eric was right behind her, and the minute I saw his eyes, I knew that he was on something. Mom, of course, was acting as if there was nothing wrong. She didn't even apologize for being late. Right away, she started talking about her date the night before, as if anyone was interested. Eric headed right for the family room, swigging down a beer I didn't see him carry in." As a sour aside, Julie added, "Mom pranced along behind me into the kitchen – right past my beautiful table – without saying a word. Honestly," she said, "I didn't know whether to laugh or cry: I'd worked so hard to make it nice for her and, as always, she didn't even notice." The Group, refrained from saying anything, knowing that Julie was not yet finished.

Swallowing hard, Julie went on. "The kids were behaving like little angels until Eric used the remote control to turn their movie off and turn to the sports channel. Sometimes," she said, exasperated, "Eric acts like a ten-year-old. Of course, Mom just sat down, expecting me to wait on her. Meanwhile, the kids started to fuss and Tom tried to calm them down." As an aside, she added, "That's the one thing that surprised me; usually the kids come running to me but, this time, Tom took charge. Now, all I wanted was to feed them so they'd go home. So I got dinner on the table as fast as possible. I was really proud of the kids. They were just wonderful, even though it was way past their dinner time. Actually, it was past all of our dinner times. So everyone came right to the table when I called. Except for Eric, who was still in the family room, swearing at the TV because his team was losing. When he finally came to the table, I could see that he was on the edge of losing it. He started getting louder and louder, complaining about the players and saying that they were all a bunch of losers. Then he looked around the table and a little voice inside me said, 'Here we go again!' That's when he slammed his can down, sloshing beer all over. He got so loud and vulgar that he scared the kids and they started to cry. Then he yelled at them to stop being sissies. Mom kept talking, oblivious to everything. Suddenly, I'd had it. In my calmest voice, I asked Eric to stop scaring the kids. It didn't help – it just made him madder, and he yelled even louder. Only now, it was at me. Tom knew it was time to remove the kids and he got up. That's when Mom finally stopped talking. She was looking directly at me with this expression on her face – like, 'you're doing it again,' as if it was all my fault."

Julie went on to describe how, for the millionth time in her life, she'd tried reasoning with Eric. But when it became obvious that he was beyond control, she knew she had to get him outside. "His aggressiveness left me no choice," Julie said. "So, I ignored my mother and ordered Eric out of the house. After asking him three times, he finally got up and bolted to the door, yelling obscenities and knocking furniture every which way. At that point, my mother screamed, 'Thanks a lot, Julie; you've just made things worse.' I knew it was too dangerous for anyone to come near him so I went into the kitchen and called the police. Then I followed the sound of Eric's voice out into the front yard where Tom was trying to talk him into calming down. But it wasn't working," she said. "Eric turned on Tom, jeering at him for being a loser and threatening him with a lawsuit if he got any closer. Tom didn't back down," Julie said proudly, "and Eric pitched his beer can at him just as the police arrived. It was just awful," she said. "All of our neighbors came out to see what was going on as the police cuffed Eric and put in him the back of the squad car. But I had to do it, just like all the other times!" she said, shamefacedly.

Familiar with this kind of public humiliation, Kate nodded. She'd started experiencing that kind of hurt, fear, and embarrassment when she was only a child. And it hadn't changed much with Ed. The others in the Group, not having been through an experience like this, could only sympathize. And that's what they did, listening carefully and trying to put themselves in Julie's place. How would they respond in a situation like this? Julie went on to say that the police took Eric to a psychiatric hospital because they thought he might hurt someone. "He's still there and I know he's still mad at me for calling the police. But as dreadful as that day went," she said, "after they'd driven off, my mother turned to me and said, 'How could you do this to us?' When I tried to explain that I was afraid he would injure someone again, all she could say was, 'You always manage to set him off – why can't you be more careful about what you say to him?'" Julie's shoulders drooped. "Sometimes I wonder," she said, "how the three of us can be in the same family." She stopped, fearfully waiting to hear what everyone would say. Would they be shocked by her family? Would they think she was just as crazy as her mother and brother? Thinking that, would they want her out of the Group? To Julie's surprise, and relief, no one thought any such thing. They were shocked of course – it was an appalling situation. But along with their surprise, Julie could see compassion on their faces. Speaking from her heart, Margaret said, "It must have really hurt when your mother said those things." Her hand flashing to cover her heart, Julie nodded. Hurt was an understatement.

Emily, knowing how much work it took to put on a party, said, "She didn't even notice how hard you worked." Marti summed it all up by saying, "In spite of all the chaos and danger, you handled everything so well. And," she added, "you didn't let your mother keep you from doing what you knew was right." All the praise was suddenly too much for Julie. Prepared to be rejected, she was instead receiving understanding and support, and from people she'd come to respect and admire. Released so unexpectedly from a lifelong fear, she burst into tears. "Oh," she sobbed, "I've never told anyone about my family before. I was afraid that if people knew about them they wouldn't want to have anything to do with me." Hearing this, Marti thought that Julie had taken a big risk with the Group, and it had worked out better than she'd ever expected. Reaching this new level of trust, Julie would now be able to turn her journey inward. To Julie she said, "I'm so proud of you for taking a chance and sharing these uncomfortable feelings with us. What was it like for you?"

Willing her tears away, Julie replied, "I can't believe that I finally have people in my life who listen, who actually hear what I have to say. I've always . . ." She stopped for a moment, unable to hold back her tears, then said, "I've always felt so alone." Tears in her own eyes, Margaret thought, Poor Julie. She's felt alone all this time.

Looking around, Julie saw that others had tears in their eyes, too. What she didn't know was that they could all relate to the feeling of not being heard, and the lonely feeling that always follows.

Marti didn't want to interrupt this moment, but with only a short time left for Julie, the therapist wanted to help her see the relationship between family catastrophe and food. Marti brought that about with, "I'm curious about how all this might have affected your food this week." This was a questions Marti asked in relation to everything, but it was the first time she'd ever directed it to Julie.

Stalling to think it over, Julie searched for an honest answer "Right after my mother and brother left, I noticed that my appetite had disappeared," she said. "So I fed the kids and Tom, but I couldn't eat a thing. The next morning when the kids wanted birthday cake for breakfast I went along with it and had a small piece, too. But, doing that really started something because I kept going back for more. All weekend long, I ate a bite here and a forkful there, until I'd eaten the whole thing. I think," Julie concluded now, "that eating kept my mind away from worrying. I know that Mom is going to do something to get even with me, I just don't know what. Believe me, it's not over!"

Pleased with Julie's evaluation, Marti asked, "Thinking about how you were feeling during this time, what do you think you were looking for?" Promptly, Julie replied, "I needed something to calm my nerves!" Marti smiled. "Did the cake do that?" she asked. "Not really," Julie said, "I don't even remember eating it. I just knew it was there and I couldn't stop thinking about it until it was gone." Marti, thrilled with Julie's increasing clarity, asked, "And after eating all of the cake, how did your body feel?"

"Terrible," Julie said. "I felt totally bloated, and I had a headache all day."

"So," Marti said, "the cake didn't do a good job of giving you what you really needed. I'm wondering, Julie, if there was something else you could have done that would have been more helpful?" Turning to the others, she asked, "Anyone have any suggestions?"

"Long soaking baths always work for me," Emily said.

"Sometimes it helps to talk about it," Margaret said. "I want you to know that you can call me anytime because I'm always home." Then Kate came up with a suggestion that surprised them all. "Watching the shopping channel takes my mind off things," she said, setting Marti up to wonder what that was all about. But, needing to keep her attention on Julie, she said, "It will be interesting to see if any of these suggestions work for you. Or, maybe you'll think of something else." Returning to Julie's original question, the therapist commented, "I wonder if you now might have an answer to why your weight came and stayed!"

Having mulled this one over a lot, Julie said, "Yes. I think that the weight, MY weight, came to protect me from rejections. If I didn't allow anyone to get really close to me, it wouldn't hurt as much when they left."

"Good for you," said Marti. "Like the rest of us, your weight didn't just show up. There's a definite reason for it being there. As you learn to protect yourself in other ways, there won't be a need for the extra weight and it will begin to come off." Suddenly, all of this was too much for Julie. Very quietly, she nodded in acknowledgment and said, "I'm finished; thank you."

A few seats away, a rattled Bobbie was trying to apply all of this to herself. She envied those who could uncover things about themselves. But how could they allow themselves to be so vulnerable in front of each other, she wondered. If it took crying in class to get her answers, Marti could count her out. Even though she'd gotten really misty during Julie's recital, crying about her own problems in class was not something she was willing to do. Recovered now from that lapse in steely reserve, she decided to go next. Having done that, she remembered that they would probably be expecting an update. Why had she ever told them about Garth and the credit card? Well, there was nothing she could do about that but explain. So Bobbie plunged ahead, saying, "Garth is on the road again so I still don't know how, or when, payment is going to be made on my account."

Going so abruptly from the vulnerable admissions of Julie to this bluntly phrased statement caught everyone off guard. Even Kate blinked. But Bobbie was moving on, trying to explain that she might be worried about nothing because maybe he'd already paid it. Then, before anyone could respond with a statement or question, she was moving on to what she hoped was a safer subject.

"Well, I discovered this week that there is something missing in my life – and it's not like I have the faintest idea what it might be. I mean, I have a nice place to live, my car is old but in good condition, I'm in a relationship, and I have a good job. So, what could be missing?" Again, before anyone might interrupt the flow, she raced on. "To tell the truth, I don't know when I'd have time for anything else, anyway." Then she took a breath. And Margaret made a comment. "It's beyond me," she said, her voice comfortingly gentle, "how you can keep up with your schedule. You're doing something every single minute of the day, from the time you get up until you crash into bed at night." Relieved that this was all that Margaret was commenting on, Bobbie was only too willing to acknowledge her hectic pace with, "On the days I work, I'm very, very busy. But I do have days off." Emily was immediately curious about this; Bobbie had never mentioned having free time before. "What do you do on your days off?" Emily asked.

Pleased at the direction in which the conversation was going, Bobbie replied, "When I'm not working extra shifts, I collapse. Some days, I'm so exhausted that I don't even get dressed." Emily waited for more. When it didn't come, she asked, "What do you do for fun?"

"Fun?" Bobbie said, visibly confused by the question. "When would I have time for that?" And, she wondered, what on earth would I do?

From this interchange Marti suspected that the cat might be out of the bag. Picking up on a key word – Time – Marti formed a question to help Bobbie associate what was missing with a lack of time. "Bobbie," she asked, "if you could have one wish, what would you wish for?" As she'd expected, Bobbie said, "Time!"

"It sounds like that's going to be a very important word for you," Marti observed. The way Bobbie tipped her head, Marti knew that she wasn't getting it and probed, "I wonder what it feels like to not have any time for yourself." Bobbie sensed the shift: Marti was bringing the conversation around to emotions. Uncomfortable now, Bobbie answered, "Tired!"

Marti, knowing that being tired is a physical condition rather than a feeling, pressed on with, "Anything else?"

"Nooooo," Bobbie replied. "Not that I can think of."

"Is it possible," Marti asked, "that when you don't have time to do the things you want, like having some fun, a part of you feels neglected – maybe even angry?"

There was no escaping the feeling stuff, Bobbie thought. Sending herself searching inside, she asked herself if there was a part of her that felt neglected. Was she angry about it? To her absolute surprise, and horror, she found herself wanting to cry. Oh no, she wailed inwardly, I can't cry. Ordering her eyes to remain dry and her throat to clear, she said, "There's no time in my life for anything but work." Then her traitorous voice wobbled, and she found herself confessing, "and I'm afraid there never will be." "What about your days off?" Marti queried. Reluctantly, Bobbie admitted, "Even when I do have extra time, it's usually too late to make a movie date or something with friends. When Garth is home, he likes to do things around the house because he's gone so much."

Marti pursued this. "Could there be a connection between not having enough time and what you said earlier about something being missing in your life?" Hearing the question, Bobbie wondered if the answer was obvious to everyone else. Well, it wasn't to her, so she said, "I guess what's missing is having enough time for myself. Time has been a problem for me all of my life. I'm never on time for anything – not even staff meetings."

Sensing that she could push a little more, Marti asked, "And where does food fit into all of this?" To Bobbie, it was as if the question had come in from left field. "Food?" she repeated. Patiently, Marti asked, "Does a lack of time affect your food in any way?" Seeing Bobbie set her chin, Marti decided to structure her next statement to make it easier. "Pick a day last week and tell us about it," she suggested.

Delighted to get a reprieve from feelings, Bobbie said, "Okay. I'll tell you about last Tuesday. The staff meeting got out late, so I only had 15 minutes for lunch. I raced down to the cafeteria for something quick, but the only thing left was macaroni and cheese – and I hate macaroni and cheese. I was starving, but before I could grab anything else, I got paged back to ER. When I got there, everyone was scrambling around, getting ready for some accident victims. I forgot about being hungry until we were finished with those patients and went into the staff room. Someone had left half a large pizza. It was like I couldn't see anything but that pizza, and I scarfed down three pieces before I even thought about it. Then I got paged for another emergency. For the next few hours, I was so busy that there wasn't time to breathe. To top it off, I couldn't even leave on time. One of the other doctors called in sick, and I had to pick up half of his shift. By the time I left, I was too tired to do anything but go to a drive-through restaurant and bring home some fried chicken." Here, Bobbie paused, hoping that Marti wouldn't pick up on what she'd just said. No such luck. "Did you eat what you really wanted, and was your body hungry when you ate it?" asked Marti.

Bobbie had to admire the skill with which Marti had led the conversation around. Knowing it was useless to try and dodge things any longer, Bobbie acknowledged that she'd been starving at lunch. "But," she said, "I was called away and couldn't eat. By the time I got to the pizza, I was starving. Did I know if that's what I wanted to eat? I haven't a clue! Was I hungry for dinner?" Stopping to remember, Bobbie thought out loud, "Logically, I had to have been, but I was so wiped out that I went on automatic pilot the minute I got in my car. I still don't know if the fried chicken is what I really wanted."

Leading Bobbie through this process, Marti heard the physician's own descriptive words "automatic pilot" and knew that she had reached a critical point. If Bobbie did not make the connection, it would be almost impossible to break through her unconscious eating at work. So, another question had to be asked. "Do you see any relationship between food and having no time for yourself?" Had either Marti or Bobbie directed a glance around the table, they would have seen it. Written all over their faces was the hope that Bobbie would be able to put it together. Slowly, Bobbie replied, "Well, it's obvious that when I don't have time, I eat on the run and I have to eat what is available – not necessarily what I want." Knowing how important it was for Bobbie to hear her own choice of words, Marti repeated, "When you don't have time?"

Pleased when Bobbie took a moment to think this over, Marti was delighted when Bobbie modified what she'd said with, "I don't take the time!" Then, amazed at what had just come out of her own mouth, Bobbie said, "Isn't that funny – until now, I always thought of time as something you have, not something that you can take." To herself, Bobbie added, Wow, where did that come from? To the rest of them, she concluded, "Which means that time is something I can take when I want or need it!"

As everyone else exhaled breaths of relief, Marti went on to tie things together. "Exactly right, Bobbie. When you don't take time to think about what you want, you have to make do with what's there. Then, when you don't eat what you want, your hunger isn't satisfied, which sends you searching for what your body wanted in the first place. And you keep eating in the hope of finding that right taste or texture. Which brings us back to unconscious eating and weight gain."

Why had it been so difficult to make this connection? Bobbie wondered. Once you looked at it, it was obvious. Aloud, she said, "I think that my environment at work has contributed more to my weight gain than I thought. In the ER, time is something you fight – not something you take. It's crisis after crisis. That means that every decision we make can mean the difference between life and death. When someone is finally out of danger, there's a kind of high that sends all of us toward the food machines. Whether our hunger is physical or not, I don't know. But everyone hits that lunch room and starts gobbling down whatever is there." Something else occurred to her. "Now that I think of it, there's always a ton of food in there." Knowing that intense feelings usually accompany that kind of stress, Marti wanted to help Bobbie become more aware of her emotions at work. So she asked, "Bobbie, can you tell us what feelings you experience when you're working through a crisis?"

Back to feelings, again, Bobbie thought. But, somehow, it seemed less threatening this time. So she said, "Well, I have to be able to think and act fast. And I have to know how to handle family and friends of the patients, too. They're going through a lot and are usually very upset." Listening, Marti was aware that the physician was describing other people's feelings, not her own. "For instance," Bobbie went on, "last night we had a 57-year-old man come in with a heart attack. He wasn't breathing, and when that happens everyone has to rush against time. Right away, I got this rush of adrenalin and started barking out orders. People were running in every direction. Test results were coming in and, in a split second, his heart stopped. Now, we have no time at all if we're going to save him. So I'm pushing everyone to work faster. We give him more medication, CPR, the paddles – the whole works. By now, the pace is a killer, and half an hour later, he died anyway. While I'm out telling the family, another emergency was coming in the door."

Observing that the physician had described her physical reactions rather than emotional, Marti knew that behind those taut muscles and increased breathing were strong feelings and that Bobbie was getting closer to discovering what they were. To get her in touch with them, Marti asked, "What are you feeling right now?" The question stopped Bobbie in her tracks: hadn't she just mentioned the adrenalin rush? Could there be more? So Bobbie listened to the pounding in her ears and reported, "My heart's racing. My breathing is increasing, too."

Noticing that Bobbie was still only describing physical reactions, Marti repeated, "So what are you feeling now?" This time, Bobbie didn't have an answer. Seeing how difficult it was for her to identify her feelings, Kate came to the rescue. "It looks like you're feeling nervous," she said. Margaret chimed in with, "How about anxious? I'm feeling anxious just listening to you."

The words hit home. "You're right," Bobbie admitted. "That's exactly how I feel."

Marti smiled and said, "Looking at how anxious you can be at work, can you see a relationship between dealing with crisis and the urge to eat?" On a roll, now, Bobbie replied, "Yes. When everything is over, I'm often still so pumped up that I could do four or five more codes without stopping. Eating gets rid of that feeling." Marti nodded. "So, eating helps you handle anxiety?" she asked. "And using food to deal with feelings is a big part of TEAM eating."

"No wonder I can't lose weight," Bobbie exclaimed. "But that's the way it is. No one can change the circumstances."

Marti was ready for this discouraging statement. "Maybe," she said, "and maybe not! One suggestion that might be helpful is to grab a few minutes every now and then to regroup." Not seeing how, Bobbie nixed it. "That's impossible when I'm on duty!" Marti continued as if she hadn't spoken. "I don't mean physically leaving the ER. But you must need to use the bathroom occasionally. So, while you're in there, relax your body by closing your eyes and taking deep breaths. Physically relaxing your body reduces anxiety. When you're tense, anxiety increases."

The simplicity of a possible truth struck Bobbie hard. "I can't believe that my work is the very thing making me gain weight," she said self-doubt and anguish in her voice. "I guess I'll give it a try because I can't leave ER; I've worked too hard to get where I am. Besides, I love my work; it's more important to me than anything else in my life."

Understanding Bobbie's dilemma, Marti said, "It's not easy to look at this, and stay with your feelings if you think the only way to comfort yourself is with food." That did it – the tears that Bobbie had so determinedly kept back came rushing out. Mortified by their silent tears slipping down her cheeks, she apologized. But Marti would have none of that. "There's nothing to apologize for. It's okay to cry," the therapist said reassuringly, "it's nature's way of releasing your feelings." Grabbing a tissue, Bobbie said she was finished and Marti asked who wanted to be next. Thinking to herself how Bob-

bie's tears expressed a vulnerability that made her more approach-
able, more human, and more connected with the rest of them, Kate
raised her hand. Not because she was enthusiastic about it being her
turn, but because she could see that Bobbie was very uncomfortable
crying in front of everyone. So, Kate jumped into the breach with,
"Ed's back!"

Little gasps could be heard around the table. Everyone had come
to feel very protective of Kate, especially when Ed was around. Kate
continued with, "The rat didn't say where he'd been, he just showed
up at work last Wednesday. He probably thought it would be easier
to face me there than alone at home." Then, aware that everyone's
eyes were riveted upon her, she sighed and forced herself to explain.

"When I saw him come through the door I actually got sick to my
stomach. It didn't get any better because he spent the rest of the day
avoiding me and kissing up to the employees. It was so disgusting
that I couldn't even eat lunch. By five o'clock, I had a world-class
headache and went home, took a few aspirin, and went straight to
bed, not caring if he came home or not. A few hours later, I heard
his key in the lock. I got up and was waiting for him when he came
into the bedroom. Before he could open his mouth, I said, 'So,
where the hell have you been?' He, of course, had the nerve to tell
me that it was none of my business. So we ended up having this
huge fight." Kate was surprised that, having admitted this, made her
feel as if she'd just gotten rid of an enormous weight – almost as if
she'd rolled a boulder off her back. This weird sort of freedom was
so unexpected that she stopped, providing Marti with the chance to
ask, "How did it feel to confront Ed?" Before thinking about her
answer, Kate was saying, "Great! In spite of all the name-calling and
shouting, it was good to finally put into words what I'd felt for so
long" She went on to say that when Ed wouldn't stop yelling, she
went downstairs and turned on the shopping channel really loud.
"Some time later when I got hungry," she said, "I fixed myself some
soup and a sandwich. And wouldn't you know that as I sat down to

eat the only thing I'd been able to swallow since breakfast, Ed walked into the kitchen!" Indignantly, she said, "He had the nerve to ask, 'Where's mine?'"

When everyone else appeared as incensed as she'd been, Kate elaborated. "I told him to fix his own. He didn't of course; he grabbed some beer out of the refrigerator and went back upstairs. An hour or two later when I got the urge to have some nachos," Kate said, "he came back downstairs before I was finished. He was so drunk that I was surprised that he could still walk. Then he saw my nachos and said, 'Someone as fat as you shouldn't eat that crap!' Maybe it was because I'd lost eight pounds while he was gone, but I came right back at him with, 'It's none of your damn business what I eat! I don't have to answer to you or anybody else.'" She stopped, tired beyond imagining until she heard a soft cheer. Surprised, she looked around to see what looked like pride on everyone's faces – for her! Their next words validated it.

"It's terrible that he said those things to you," said Emily, unable to envision anyone – not even her mother – being so outspoken.

"Has he always talked to you that way?" asked Julie.

"Yes," Kate said, "in high school whenever I put on weight, he was the first one to mention it. But in the past few years he's gotten downright mean about it." Then it was Marti's turn. "What have you done in the past when he verbally attacked you?" For a minute, Kate was speechless. Hearing the words "verbal attacks" out loud somehow made it seem so serious. She could feel the heat rise in her neck and face. Flippantly, she replied, "I considered the source!"

Perceptively, Marti asked, "What are you feeling right now?" Brought back so unexpectedly to the here and now, Kate was flustered enough to say, "Furious!" And she was. Her eyes suddenly ablaze, she said, "And I'm not only mad at Ed, I'm mad at me for putting up with it for all these years. I'm his wife after all! He's supposed to love and protect me, not put me down. I don't know why he does it to me; what can I do to stop him?" Wanting Kate to see the whole picture, Marti asked, "Why are you accepting all of the responsibility for fixing this situation? Isn't Ed responsible for what he does and says?"

Uneasily, Kate considered, then admitted, "It's easier to do everything myself." What she didn't say was that if she acknowledged that Ed did have a part in it, she would then have to admit that she was helpless to get him to change his ways. That left her with only one alternative, and she wasn't ready, yet. Thinking it over, she said, "Ed doesn't think that he has a problem – it's ME who has one! So," she said, throwing up her hands, "the situation is hopeless." There, she'd said it. Then, all by itself, her mouth opened once more and she heard herself voicing the rest. "I guess my only option is to divorce him." With those words it was as if all of the air suddenly drained from the room. Into this emptiness flowed her fear – and everyone else's: Give up – walk away – divorce?

This was, Marti knew, a good example of black and white thinking. The problem with this kind of extremist view was that it left no room for a person to consider, evaluate, compromise, or negotiate. Kate's word "divorce" came not from any sort of choice, but as a reaction to feeling helpless. Marti addressed that, saying, "Kate, you have more than two choices. It's not either stay and take Ed's abuse or divorce him!" Kate clearly did not believe this. Her next words were almost a dare. "Like what?" she asked

Marti met the challenge by saying, "Ed might change in response to a difference in you – just as Julie's children did once they understood what she expected of them. They realized that she meant it when she said it was bedtime, so they stopped challenging her and obeyed. You've only just started letting Ed know how you expect to be treated." Kate didn't see the relationship at all. "If I can't get Ed to listen to what I say, how can I change his behavior?" she queried.

Patiently, Marti explained, "This isn't about changing Ed. It's about you – and everyone else in Group – deciding how you expect to be treated by others, saying it out loud to those who need to hear it, and sticking to it. It's only fair to let the important people in your lives know what you expect from them. At that point, they can choose to change... or not!"

Dimly, this began to make sense to Kate and she stopped objecting. "You mean," she said, "I can't blame Ed for not doing what I want if I haven't told him what that is?"

"You've got it!" Marti said. "And Kate, you've already begun to do that."

"Okay," Kate said. "But what do I do next?"

Pleased at the breakthrough, Marti said, "Before you do anything, you may want to consider how you feel about his drinking, his disappearances, and his abusive language. Alcoholism is a progressive disease. As it gets worse, so does a drinker's anger, tension, blaming, and demeaning words. And even after people have stopped drinking, they can still continue their abusive behaviors if they haven't addressed the issues that led to these conditions."

Marti's description of Ed as an alcoholic sent the pit of Kate's stomach plummeting. No one had even suggested that before. Was he an alcoholic? Timorously, she asked "Do you really think Ed's an alcoholic?" Marti's reply was firm. "Yes, I do." When Kate looked around and saw everyone nodding in agreement, she nearly burst into tears. Of course, Ed was an alcoholic; somewhere inside she'd known it for years. Then, with denial falling in shards around her, Kate had to take control: she'd change the locks tomorrow. But what if he knocked the doors down? And what about the business? How could she run it by herself? What would she tell the employees? What would customers say? Stopped in her tracks by unknown answers, she said, "If Ed would just stop drinking, it would solve everything!"

Understanding that Kate had returned to her old, helpless way of thinking, Marti said, "If anything is going to happen in a positive way, you have to change your focus from Ed to yourself. That means that you are going to have to decide for yourself what you want in this relationship. Once it is clear to you, tell it in no uncertain terms to Ed and see if he wants the same kind of relationship you do. If he does, then ask if he is willing to make the changes necessary for that kind of relationship to develop. If he chooses to try, we can establish ways for it to be successful. If he continues to drink and be abusive, then you will need to continue to make decisions based upon his behavior." Looking at Kate, Marti could see protests forming. So she continued, "The good news is that you've already taken that first step. Others are coming, and you will take them, too. All of them together will eventually lead to change." Relieved that Marti was not scolding or blaming her for anything, Kate sagged into her chair. "It's going to take time, isn't it?" Marti nodded. "Change doesn't happen overnight," she said. Then it was time to move on. Turning to Margaret and Emily, Marti asked, "Who wants to go next?"

Margaret raised her hand. "I'm sort of in the same spot Bobbie was in," she began. "I haven't been able to figure out what's missing in my life, either. Especially because I'm already doing everything I think is important. Yet, I have this feeling that I want something more – I just don't know what it is." Directing her remarks to the younger women, she explained, "I dropped out of college to get married, which is what we did in those days – from childhood, we were taught that girls grew up to be wives and mothers. College was important because it provided opportunities to meet young men with good futures. As soon as we found the right one, we dropped out and took jobs to support their ambitions.

"Looking back," Margaret said, "we struggled a lot those first years, even though Bob's schooling expenses were covered because he was a veteran. The only spending money we had came from what I made as a secretary, but we were so happy. Then, he graduated and went on to law school. About the time he joined a law firm, we had a baby. The timing couldn't have been better! After a few years, he was promoted to junior partner and that's when my life changed again. Suddenly with a baby and a toddler, I was expected to join the 'right' committees and clubs, and we were expected to go to events considered important by the senior partners and their wives. Added to that were the children and all of their activities. I swear, most of my time was spent in a car, going to and coming from somewhere." Remembering all that activity, Margaret had to smile. "In all honesty, I loved it," she said. "And I continue to enjoy the people and events that are important to Bob's career." Sensing that, maybe, the younger women found this hopelessly old-fashioned, she hastened to add, "It's not like Bob's told me that I have to do any of those things, and I wouldn't let any of them get in the way of my time with my granddaughter. I guess what's confusing is that I have everything that should make me happy and fulfilled but, somehow, it doesn't seem to be enough anymore. Something is out-of-place, or missing, and I wish I knew what it was."

Bobbie felt renewed by this recital. Having a career instead of a husband and children solved most of life's problems, she thought. Julie, on the other hand, regarded Margaret's life as ideal: how wonderful it would be, she thought, to have a rich, powerful man taking you to the opera and champagne dinners with the most important people in town. Whenever Margaret mentioned Devon, it struck Julie hard. Life would have been so different if her grandmother had half the love and devotion Margaret has for Devon, she thought. To Margaret, she said, "Every child ought to have a grandmother like you." Touched, Margaret replied, "I wish everyone felt that way!" It caught everyone by surprise. To answer their unspoken question, Margaret explained that her son and his ex-wife felt that she was overprotective. "But maybe I wouldn't be if I saw them being more careful," she said. Marti picked up on that. "Sounds like you are concerned about Devon's welfare."

Folding and unfolding her hands, Margaret finally answered. "My son and Cheryl do things that I consider downright reckless, like letting Devon go to strangers' houses to play. They even drop her off at birthday parties without knowing the parents or who else is going to be there." Emily was confused about this. "Do you mean they should know not only the kids but all of the adults who are going to be there?" she asked. Margaret was adamant in her reply. "Yes," she said, "they should know exactly who's going to be there. But, then, I've always been protective of her since the day she was born. Lately, I find myself worrying about her all the time."

Hearing this, Emily couldn't help but apply Margaret's concerns to her own children. She didn't always check, either. Should she? At the same time, Julie was wondering, too; should she worry more about the other families who used her children's daycare? Marti wanted to help Margaret identify the source of her concerns, so she asked, "Are you saying that your fears are increasing? Why? What danger are you perceiving?"

Margaret seemed not to know. "There's nothing in particular, I just don't want anything bad to happen to her," she replied. "She's at such a vulnerable age; so trusting and innocent that she'll go anywhere with anyone." Just talking about this was taking its toll on Margaret. "I'm just afraid," she whispered, wringing her fingers, "that if her parents aren't more careful, she's going to get hurt." Knowing that this was the time to persist, Marti asked, "How do you know this?"

Here it was, thought Margaret; the right moment to bring everything out in the open. Taking a deep breath, she said, "Because I was her age when I was sexually abused." Around her, everyone froze. Margaret? This loving, kind woman, had been abused? Their hearts sinking, each member of the Group found herself experiencing an age-old sense of horror. But Margaret, having finally told them, found herself feeling relieved. At the same time, she was thinking how big a risk it had been to reveal her secret. What was everyone thinking? Feeling shame and humiliation, she couldn't continue. Into the vacuum of uneasy silence came Marti's concerned voice. "Do you need a few minutes?" she asked. Taking a few more deep breaths, Margaret said, "No." She went on. There was no turning back now.

"My parents had taken me to spend the night at my aunt and uncle's house. After we were asleep, my uncle came into my room and climbed into my bed. I didn't remember that, or anything that followed it, until a couple of years ago when, out of the blue, perfectly normal things started triggering these horrible memories. After trying everything to get rid of them, I went into therapy and talked about that night for the first time. Then I started to remember other things, like my parents' reaction when I told them. You see, because my uncle was my father's brother, I'm not sure that anyone really believed me. At any rate, nothing was ever said after that. I never saw either my aunt or my uncle again. I remember that my parents started arguing all the time. I also remember that during the following year, I went from thin to plump, and then to fat. Maybe I wouldn't have even noticed except that the kids at school teased me about it. Then my parents divorced and that was worst of all." Clearly upset now, Margaret finished by saying, "And all of it was my fault. If I hadn't been abused, my parents would probably still be together."

This was such an old, deep wound that Marti was careful to say just the right thing. "What happened with your parents is not your fault. They had their own reasons for not being able to work things out, and it had nothing to do with you. You were only five when these awful things happened, and unfortunately there was no one there willing to talk to you about it. Children don't have many tools to deal with this kind of thing. Without someone to talk to, you were left with a lot of frightening feelings, and weird feelings in your body that you didn't know what to do with. Because children are dependent upon their parents to validate what is and is not important, when no one responds to their abuse, children internalize that the experience is unimportant. Eventually, they act as if it never happened. But, when five-year-olds feel icky on the inside, they begin to scan their environment for a reason why. The only thing that seems reasonable to them is that there is something wrong with their body. So what you remember as a child is feeling gross and uncomfortable in your body, but not why you felt that way."

"I remember," Margaret said, reaching for a tissue. Marti waited before continuing with, "You also remember kids teasing you because of your weight, reinforcing your belief that there was something wrong with it."

Crying, Margaret nodded and said, "I just felt so empty – like I could never get full. I couldn't stop eating. Although, not long ago, I looked at pictures and I wasn't as fat as I'd thought."

"So was food a way of comforting yourself when there were no other ways to get comfort?" asked Marti.

"Yes," Margaret replied, "I guess so . . ."

Marti asked, "Is it possible that when the memories and feelings began to return two years ago, you went back to the old ways of dealing with the pain?"

"Maybe," said Margaret, thinking back.

Going on, Marti proposed, "Maybe some of your need to protect Devon is related to a need to care for that abused little girl inside of you." Margaret, having never considered that before, began to cry. What Marti said was true. Margaret then realized how much she had been worrying about her own little girl deep inside. She'd been hurting for so long. Softly, she said, "There's no way to keep her safe!"

Having made an important connection between her abuse and her weight, Marti knew it was essential to guide Margaret toward more accurate ways of dealing with her feelings. She continued with, "It must be hard to accept that your granddaughter can't be protected every minute of the day. But food isn't what you need to protect the little girl inside or yourself now. What else would make you feel safe and comforted?" she asked.

"I don't know," Margaret said, softly, through her tears, "food has always been my friend!"

Sadness filled the room; everyone empathized with the feelings that came from eating certain foods for comfort. Until now, it seemed there had been no other way. Kate chimed in, "Food is the one thing you can trust!" Emily agreed. "It's always there when you need it!" she said.

"Well it works for a while, anyway," Margaret admitted. "But I can see now that the feelings will never go away as long as I smother them with food."

Marti agreed. "Food is a temporary solution that diverts us momentarily from our feelings. But the goal shouldn't be to find a distraction to escape those emotions," she said. "The goal is to find more accurate ways of dealing with them. You know, Margaret, as you continue to find other ways to help you cope with your feelings, food will become a less important source of soothing yourself." Just beginning to absorb what she'd just learned, Margaret wiped away her tears and turned to Emily. "It's your turn," she said.

"I never thought I could do it," Emily began, "but I've been eating what I really want in front of everyone I know. However, I was scared to death that when I did, I'd gain weight. So, although we're not supposed to be weighing ourselves, I got on the scales this week. When I found that I'd gained a couple of pounds, I felt I had no choice but to go back to diet foods." Having said that, Emily took a wary peek at Marti. Shocked into asking another question, Julie asked, "And what happened?" Abashed, Emily said, "I couldn't eat it."

"You couldn't eat it?" echoed Kate.

Her voice defeated, Emily replied, "No. It tasted terrible. I guess I've gotten so used to eating real food that the diet stuff tasted like reconstituted cardboard. I wonder how I ever survived on that stuff. But I have to tell you, the biggest surprise is that it didn't give me the same feeling it always gave me before. In the past, it made me believe that everything was going to be okay. You see," she explained, "it used to be that I was willing to deprive myself for a while because

I thought I'd be losing weight right away. That gave me a feeling of control – but not anymore." Relating this to the assignment, she added, "So I guess what's missing in my life is the belief that losing weight will solve everything. It's pretty terrifying to know that's not true. I guess what I'm saying," she said, "is that I can't diet anymore."

Hearing her voice rise with every word, everyone knew that Emily wasn't kidding. They understood that having reached the point of facing the demise of an old belief, she felt bereft. Kate broke in. "I hate to admit it," she confessed, "but a couple of weeks ago I got upset because I wasn't losing fast enough and I thought seriously about rejoining one of those diet programs. But then I had to admit that I just couldn't go back." Julie followed up with, "But you can't get away from diets and dieting. When a friend at work went on the newest one and dropped five pounds in a week, I was really tempted. Except the quick and mindless isn't the answer for me anymore – I'm not turning back, either." Marti, knowing that it was important for Emily to acknowledge her feeling about this loss, asked, "What does it feel like to know that you don't have the diet option anymore?" she asked.

Thoughtfully, Emily said, "It scares me; if this doesn't work, I'm going to be stuck with…" Pointing at herself, she finished, "this body forever." Marti shook her head. "It's not easy to give up old beliefs and behaviors, especially when you haven't assimilated new ones to replace them. You might be feeling a sense of loss over letting the old ways go, even if they didn't work." This sounded like grieving to Bobbie, and she brought that up. "Are you suggesting that we might actually be mourning the loss of those old diets?" Marti nodded. "Those feelings can be overwhelming at times. But if you let that stop you from going on, feeling overwhelmed will be replaced with feeling scared. Then you will be stuck again." To Emily, this made sense. "I guess," she said, "we all have a lot to think about this week." With that, Marti picked up their next assignment. "This next week you will begin to look at your current lifestyle to see what is, and isn't, working for you." Uneasy because she still didn't feel that she had a handle on being as aware as she should be, Bobbie asked, "You mean we're finished with eating consciously?"

"Definitely not!" said Marti. "No matter what we do from now on, it will be in addition to eating consciously. Starting this week, each of you will begin thinking about creating a lifestyle that will support losing weight and keeping it off. That means you will be looking for ways to more accurately take care of your other hungers, too." Marti handed out their packets.

CHAPTER SIX

I'd Rather Be Fat Than Exercise!!

Week Thirteen: Responding More Accurately to Other Hungers

*N*O ONE WAS FINDING IT EASY to push beyond analyzing their relationships to food to look at other things, mainly because they'd just gotten used to their new relationship with food; and to making choices on what to eat and what not to eat based upon how the food made their bodies feel. It was an empowering experience. But they were asked to extend the methodical, careful examination they had been giving to food to other areas of their lives. Broadening awareness was difficult. Each was constantly asking herself: what do I want? How can I change things to make it better for myself?

As Marti had come to expect, each member of the group was beginning to see that one of her main focuses in life had been to make other people happy. Now as they began taking time to examine everything around them, the women began feeling disloyal in transferring this attention, even for a moment or two, to themselves. For Bobbie, it was especially difficult to be looking at her food and at the same time other areas of her life. It was still hard to take time for herself. With more things to do, she felt like she needed to take more time to do it all. And, for Bobbie, time was a precious, and scarce, commodity.

With Garth away on a two-week sales trip, Bobbie forced herself to do the assignment calling on them to evaluate their usual routines for caring for their bodies. The eye exam and physical exam had been easy, of course, because hospital personnel were required to have regular checkups. What bothered her was having to judge the superficial stuff: make-up, clothing, and hairstyle. What hairdo? She just pulled hers back into a ponytail or bun. And what about the colors in her wardrobe? Did she like the fabrics? How about the textures and styles? I mean, Bobbie fumed, I have more important things to do. But the questions must have stirred some sort of interest because she found herself thinking about them.

Julie, on the other hand, had been completely caught up in the exercise. She went so far as to ask a friend who sold cosmetics to give her a make-over. Upon seeing how this season's new shades and techniques altered her appearance, Julie had actually bought the starter kit. Her next surprise came when she found how easy make-up was to apply. By the time the next Group meeting came along, she'd gotten pretty good at doing it. When everyone loved it, she had to admit that she was pleased, too. Then, in the twelfth week, Margaret took the plunge. She showed up not only with a new hair style, but also a new color, everyone shared her excitement. "I knew it was time to try something new," she announced. "I was bored with my natural salt-and- pepper." Laughingly, she confessed, "I don't know who was happier with the change, my hairdresser or me!"

Over the last month, Emily had complained about having no energy. It didn't seem to matter what she ate or how much she slept, she was tired all of the time. At first, she thought it had to do with working too hard not that there was anything she could do about that! So she doubled up on vitamins, hoping they would help. It didn't, and she found herself not wanting to do anything. Nothing seemed to be helping, not even Group. What difference did it make if you liked the colors of your clothes or not when the point was that they were too big!

Sometimes, though, Emily was aware of a new voice inside yelling and screaming at her that she wasn't doing enough. "You're bad," the voice accused. "You'll never get anywhere!" To quiet the voice, she'd allowed a friend at work to give her a manicure in the hopes of making her feel better. It hadn't. She was too tired to do this past week's assignment, too. It called for them to move their bodies, and she hated exercise of all kinds. Emily wondered what Kate would have said about it, but Kate hadn't been in class for the past three weeks. The messages she'd left on Marti's answering machine said that she was leaving town for awhile. While Marti told the Group this, she didn't tell them that the messages worried her. Not that Kate was going to be away, but that she had not sounded at all like someone who was leaving on a vacation.

The last session Kate had attended had been very emotional for her, and everyone saw how uncomfortable that had made her. Marti wondered if her leaving had something to do with a need to get away from the feelings she'd experienced. Whether that was true or not, Marti couldn't help but feel excitement and joy over all the wonderful changes happening to everyone else, despite her concern about Kate. In fact, it was amazing, she thought, how much each of them was changing, inside and out! Two weeks before, Marti had given them a new assignment. They were to ask themselves: Are you surrounded with colors you like? Is everything organized to help YOU? Do you like the furniture? Atmosphere? Do you like how the rooms look? How would you change things to make them better?

Reporting back last week, Margaret had said that, until the assignment, the only part of the house she'd ever considered hers was the kitchen. "I always felt that the rest belonged to the family," she'd explained. "When my sons left home, I continued thinking of their rooms as theirs. But the assignment brought to mind that, although Donnie is back in his old room now, the other bedroom isn't being used and could belong to me. So I gave all of my oldest son's furniture to a thrift store. Then, for the rest of the week, I kept going into it to dream about what I would like to do with it."

When it had been Emily's turn, she'd told them about the manicure first. Everyone noticed that, although she tried to appear pleased, she really wasn't. Then, in a rush, she'd said that she was happy with her house and furnishings, but not her office. She was still, she related, figuring out what needed to be done. Julie had been next and, thrilled with what she'd accomplished, she told them about going back to something she'd been putting off for years. "Tom almost dropped dead when I told him that I was going to start cleaning out the piles of stuff we've accumulated in the garage," she said. "But when he saw that I was serious, he went out and bought a sheet of heavy plywood and built a platform up on the rafters so we could store what we wanted to keep. There's still a lot to do," she acknowledged. "This weekend I only got down to the potty chair and baby clothes. But at least I've started."

Only Bobbie had shown real distress over what she'd learned through the exercise. "I realized," she said, "that everything about my condo annoys me. Maybe, that's why I sleep so much. You see," she explained, "I've not had time to decorate." When Marti asked what she could do about that, Bobbie replied,"I can't afford to decorate the whole thing, but I'd be happy with getting the bedroom done. With a comfortable chair or chaise lounge I could relax and read. Maybe, I ought to put a TV in there, too. Then I could change into something comfortable at the end of a shift, put my feet up, and not fall asleep." There was a problem, though. Bobbie admitted to not knowing what style of furniture to buy, or how to arrange it. "My mother would be only too glad to do it for me," she said. "But she'd just take over and do what she wanted." Others heard a hint of rebellion in her voice.

Knowing her own mother's tendencies, Emily knew how Bobbie

felt and was especially sympathetic. So she spoke up, along with everyone else, to give Bobbie some suggestions; everything from looking at a variety of home decorating magazines to volunteering the names of their favorite stores and salespersons. "It always helps me," Margaret said, "take time to visualize what I want." Seeing Bobbie appear grateful for their suggestions, Marti was thinking that she'd taken a dozen groups through this same process and they never failed to impress her with their determination to make the changes once they'd been identified. When you know you have the support of those around you, she thought, you can do anything! Everyone finds a way to express her own individuality in the safety of an accepting, supporting group.

* * * * *

Kate was back. What a surprise, Marti thought. No phone call. No message. Just, here she was! And quieter than usual. Actually, the others were pretty quiet, too. What was going on here? Marti wondered. Did it have to do with the movement assignment? Like other groups before them, they may have misinterpreted the directions.

Margaret voiced her objections first. Typically, she was gentle in her appraisal, starting out by saying, "The movement assignment really confused me. I didn't know what to do, so I didn't do it. Did you really want us to exercise?" Then, her moderate tone disappearing, she said more firmly, "I've never been athletic and I hate exercise classes. It doesn't feel good to jump up and down. And the music is always too loud." She paused there for a moment, then added, "Besides, I feel out of place. The instructors are so young, and have such perfect bodies." Now, what Margaret was not saying was that she'd never actually taken an exercise class. Still, she went on. "There are mirrors everywhere, and there isn't enough space in the locker rooms to change your clothes." Everyone understood what she meant, even if she didn't say it: there was never any privacy, so when you showered or changed your clothes, everybody saw everything. Now, Margaret pleaded. "Please don't make me do it!" Kate having not looked in her book for three weeks, gasped. "Were we supposed to join a gym or something?" she asked.

With every group, the thirteenth week brought the same misunderstanding. So Marti was very clear when answering the question. "No!" she said. "This assignment was not about exercise. It was about how it feels to move your body. Movement is different from exercise. Our bodies were designed to be in motion. They weren't designed to sit behind a desk or steering wheel or on a couch watching TV for long periods of time. When we don't move, we get tired. When we're tired, we need to stretch and move to increase circulation, release tension, and energize ourselves." Looking around, Marti saw that she was not selling this concept and needed to explain further.

"Often," she tried again, "we interpret feeling tired as being hungry and we eat, when all along all our body really needs is a little walk or a stretch. So this isn't about exercising to burn up calories, it's about moving around to feel better." Seeing that they still needed some convincing, Marti said, "Shifting positions, or walking around every now and then, makes sense when you remember that humans were not designed to stay in one position for any length of time. The truth is that if primitive man had just sat around, he would have died from starvation, or been eaten by predators." Margaret grinned at that. So did everyone else, relieved not only by the humor, but because Marti didn't expect them to join a gym.

Not wanting them to miss the point, Marti said, "Let's try something. Right there in your chair, find a position that's comfortable." When they did, she said, "Now, hold it for two minutes without moving anything but your eyelids." Humoring her, everyone did as they were told. One minute passed. A minute-and-a-half. But another ten seconds and Bobbie began feeling as if she was strapped to the chair. Impatiently, she said, "How much longer?" While she was the only one to say it out loud, the other four were wondering the same thing. Who would have suspected that it would be so irritating to consciously maintain a position for such a short length of time? Fortunately, Marti was counting the last seconds aloud. "Twenty more," she was saying. "Nineteen... ten... five... and finally, OK, time's up."

Even though everyone felt a little silly, they groaned with relief. To Marti's amusement, they then moved. After they'd finished sagging, stretching, yawning, and sighing, Marti laughed. "OK," she asked. "what's the first thing you did when I said that time was up?" Emily replied, "We all moved."

"How did that feel?" asked Marti. Bobbie answered with, "I was relieved because I didn't know how long I'd be able to hold still." Julie's only comment was that it "felt good."

Marti moved in to hammer the point home. "So, when you've been sitting in the same position for some time and think you need something to eat, maybe your body is telling you to move instead. Now, do you see the difference between movement and exercise?"

Margaret, wanting to make sure she'd gotten it right, asked, "So you mean that all you wanted was for us to move around?"

"Yes," Marti answered, "we wanted you to notice how you felt after you moved. For example, if you were sitting and you got up and walked, what did your body feel like?" That seemed to be worth thinking about, for everyone fell silent. Marti broke in by asking, "What's going on?"

Bobbie was the first to respond. "I move around a lot at work. At the end of my shift, I'm so tired that the thought of doing anything else is beyond me. I can't see that walking a little will make me feel less tired." Emily had a different objection. "I can see me walking the extra distance when I'm wearing pants. But when I'm wearing a dress or skirt, and pantyhose, it gets too uncomfortable." Margaret added, "I was trying to imagine walking without getting sweaty. I hate feeling sticky all over. Besides, I end up with blisters no matter what shoes I wear." Hearing that they had again jumped to the conclusion that she'd wanted them to exercise, Marti decided to take a different approach. Standing, she walked to the chalkboard and wrote:

I'm too tired.
I'm not wearing the right clothes.
I hate to feel sweaty.
I don't have the right shoes.

Then Marti drew a straight, horizontal line. Pointing to it, she said, "Movement is on a continuum. Exercise and sports are at one end." She wrote "exercise/sports" at the end of the line. "But, what we're talking about is all the way on the other end. We've been conditioned to think that the only things that count are aerobics classes, tennis, or some other sport. But, any movement counts even walking five extra feet. So, when you read your assignment, you jumped to the conclusion that we meant for you to be way over there at the end of the continuum. But the movement we're talking about is way over here." At the far left of her chalk line, she made a large X.

X _____ exercise/sports

"Some of you," she assured them, "will never choose to be in a formalized exercise program or sport. You will just be moving when your body needs it, doing activities you enjoy. Others of you, however, may eventually find yourself wanting to be even more active because it makes your body feel good. Here is how that might develop." Marti noticed that everyone was paying close attention, but she sensed that they were still suspicious. "You start with a few extra steps and notice how it feels," she continued. "If it feels good, you may want to take a few more steps. Pretty soon, you've walked ten feet. Then you're buying shoes that feel better when you walk. This encourages you to keep walking. Then you find that your walk becomes half a block, then a block, then two. At that point, you may decide to buy something more comfortable to wear. That prompts you to walk more often because it your body feels better walking with looser clothing. After a while, you're walking a mile. Then two miles. And you're looking forward to these walks because you feel lighter less stressed. And you have more energy. Now, walking has become a part of your life. Not because it's exercise you are supposed to do, but because you know how it feels in your body not to do it. It feels better to walk!" Looking around, Marti caught a glance from each person telling her that she had finally gotten through. Whether they did it or not remained up to them. Marti realized how difficult it was to turn thoughts into actions, especially when it involved moving the body. Then she turned to Margaret, who still had time to tell about what else had happened during the week.

Feeling more enthusiastic now, Margaret described where she was with her newly- requisitioned room. "I still don't know what I'm going to use it for," she said, "but it's not going to even faintly resemble a bedroom. And the color will be something light and airy." Everyone smiled at the eagerness with which she was saying this. "I'm planning to furnish it with old-fashioned rattan and wicker furniture: I just love it because it's so feminine." Her voice growing almost dreamy, Margaret said, "I think I'll put a small TV in there, too; it will be more cozy in there because all the other rooms are so big." But then, almost as if she was shocked at hearing what she'd just said, she jerked back to reality. "What I need from all of you," she said, her voice grounded now, "is to tell me that I'm not crazy for wanting this."

Seeing that she'd surprised them, Margaret said, "Well, when I said something to Bob, he got a little irritated. I wasn't expecting that because he's never denied me anything. In fact, he scolds me for not buying more for myself. But my excitement about this project caught him off-guard. When he found out that I'd given away the old furniture without telling him, he said it wasn't at all like me. And that's true," Margaret said. "I'm usually not that excited about anything." The upshot, she went on to say, was that she felt like she might be doing something wrong. For the first time, she told Bob how she felt. "I said that I was just realizing that I live in a beautiful house, but there's no place in it just for me."

"What did he say to that?" queried Julie. Margaret replied, "He didn't say anything, at first. But he looked as if I'd struck him. When he got his voice back, he said, 'What are you talking about? The whole house is yours, and you have it all to yourself all day!' I went on to explain that I'd furnished the house for him and the boys, and that if I'd been decorating just for me, it would have had a totally different look. And that's why I wanted someplace in it that's just mine where I can do whatever I want." Bobbie spoke up. "What was his reaction?" she asked.

In front of their eyes, Margaret's face grew drawn. Her voice, up until now sounding as it always did, was suddenly discouraged. "He said it was OK if it was all that important to me," Margaret said. "But it was like he gave in without really understanding how I feel. Then, he left the room without another word. Later that day, he questioned me again. He'd gone into freezer for ice. Finding seven pints of ice cream in there, he said that he didn't get it; first I'd told him that I wanted to lose weight, and then he finds ice cream in the freezer. He asked, 'What kind of diet are you on, anyway?' And that's when I started getting mad. I surprised both of us because I came right back with an answer. 'I'm supposed to eat whatever my body is hungry for including ice cream.' I didn't say any more than that," Margaret said. "I wanted to tell him it was none of his business, but I didn't want to hurt his feelings. Then he said, 'This is the damndest diet I ever heard of.' And off he went to his office." Margaret sighed. "If he'd asked, I would have told him that the ice cream had been there for weeks and I hadn't touched a bite of it. I just wanted to know that it was there if I wanted it!"

Marti was very pleased. "Good for you, Margaret, for not letting questions make you doubt what you are doing." Julie was sympathetic. "Maybe he was cranky because he's been working too hard."

"Yes, he does work a lot," Margaret said. "When he comes home, everything's always been the same until now. I've always run the house and raised the boys around his schedule. And that brings up something else," she said. "He just had a physical and our doctor told him that he had to start cutting back on his hours. That means that he'll probably be home a lot more. Is he going to be questioning everything I do from now on?" Seeing Margaret's eyes tighten, Marti asked, "What feelings are coming up right now?"

"By not wanting to know more, or allowing me to explain, it's like he's questioning my judgment," Margaret replied. "Doesn't it count that I raised two boys, ran the house, and entertained his friends and partners? Why would he question me like that?"

"How did it feel when that happened?" asked Marti. Tearfully, Margaret replied, "Like I don't count. As if what I say and want isn't important!"

In that instant, Margaret let the Group see how she really felt about herself. No wonder, Marti thought, that she's had such a difficult time communicating with other members of her family: she automatically assumes that what she has to say is unimportant especially to her husband. But Marti questioned whether this was actually true. "Has Bob ever said that you were unimportant? Or that your opinions didn't matter?" she asked. Margaret had to admit that he hadn't. Her voice neutral, Marti asked, "Then where did this belief come from?" Margaret, somewhat at a loss, replied, "I don't know, but I've always felt it." Wanting to get to the bottom of this, Marti inquired, "You've always felt this with Bob or everyone?"

That took some thought. After a short pause, Margaret said, "With everyone, I guess." With that established, Marti said, "It must be hard to communicate when you feel like whatever you say isn't going to matter anyway." The truth of that statement brought Margaret to tears. "Maybe that's why I feel like no one really knows me," she said.

Guessing that this statement reflected a feeling that was somehow connected to food, Marti wanted Margaret to identify the emotion she was experiencing right then. So she asked, "What feelings are coming up right now?" Margaret looked down into her lap. "Sadness," she said. "Loneliness!" Then she followed with, "I think I've felt that way all of my life. Perhaps more in the last few years; I just thought it was the 'empty nest' syndrome." Now Marti asked, "Is that feeling in any way connected to the abuse you experienced at five?" asked Marti.

For Margaret, the question initiated the strangest thing. Suddenly, the puzzle pieces of her life began falling into place. "I think so," she said, her words more rapid, now. And lighter. "But," she qualified, "I don't know how."

This, Marti knew, was a pivotal moment. Careful to guide rather than lead Margaret along the path to further self-enlightenment, Marti said, "Looking at what you went through, I can see how loneliness would become a key component. You were a very young child who had gone through a traumatic experience. With no one to talk to, and no one to soothe and comfort you, you were left all alone to deal with everything by yourself. Naturally, you'd feel lonely." Marti's words reawakened the confusion and fear of so many years ago and Margaret started to cry. Everything Marti said was so true; no one had ever explained what had happened, nor comforted her. But Marti wasn't finished following this line of reasoning. "Margaret," she said, "do you see a connection between what I've just described and food?"

In this class, this was a perfectly logical question, but it came as a surprise to Margaret all the same. Into her mind's eye came a picture of herself crossing the kitchen floor, going to the refrigerator, opening the freezer door and reaching inside for... ! "Yes," she replied. "And it's ice cream."

Marti wanted to stand up and yell, "AHA!" But, even this close, there was another question that had to be asked so she could be sure. So she asked, "Margaret, is it possible that, there is a connection between your weight and the abuse and the loneliness you felt after – and since – the abuse?"

Everyone saw it – a fleeting expression on Margaret's face, as if she'd just been illuminated by an internal light. Having occasionally seen this transformation at the hospital when patients received long-awaited news, Bobbie knew it to be a moment of truth. Marti knew it too, and she knew that Margaret had just added another piece to the puzzle. She could hear the change in Margaret's voice as she said, "I guess maybe I've not realized how overpowering my loneliness has been for me." Mulling this over in her mind, she said, as if to herself, "So, I wasn't ever physically hungry for ice cream. What I needed was the comfort of an old, trusted friend I could count on to be there when I wanted it. Isn't that amazing!"

Witnessing this, the others were speechless. Would their answers come in like form? Swiftly, like Margaret's, and blindingly true? For a moment everyone just sat there, sharing Margaret's reality, inspired by her victory over forces that had seemed unbeatable. Smiling, they sat. Quiet, but filled with excitement. It was in the spirit of this that Julie volunteered to be next.

Reflecting in Margaret's glow of success, Julie announced her pleasure in having found time every day just for herself. It came, she said, after putting the children to bed. "At first," she explained, "with plenty to do around the house I felt a lot of guilt taking even the 45 minutes I allotted." But then came an unexpected bonus. Those 45 minutes of relaxation were apparently affecting her sleep because she was waking up feeling far more rested than she had in years.

"That's not unusual," Marti said, "Everyone requires time to unwind both physically and mentally. Sometimes," she pointed out, "after a hectic day of doing things for everyone else, you fall into bed exhausted. Then, after a few hours of deep sleep, you wake up to spend the rest of the night wishing you could go back to sleep. That's because your mind is still in overdrive. By taking waking time to let your body rest, you give your mind a chance to slow down, too." While Julie seemed pleased to hear that her conclusion was right, it became obvious while Marti was talking that her mind was on other things. This was confirmed when she pulled a square envelope from her purse.

"I brought this along because I wanted to get your reaction to what my mother is up to now," she said, adding, "When Tom read it, he said that he was glad she was my mother, not his." Clearing her throat, she read:

To my only daughter,
You haven't returned any of my calls, so I decided to
write. I guess you must be feeling pretty bad about what
happened, and you should! None of this would have
occurred if you hadn't yelled at Eric. Couldn't you see that
he was pretty down after losing his job? He really needed
your support. But naturally, everything had to be your
way! Calling the police again really was the icing on the
cake. I'll never be able to face your neighbors again!
I know that Tom was behind it all. I wish he would mind
his own business. All I've ever wanted is for the three of us
to get along, but unless you stop listening to him and stand
up for your family, that will never happen!
Mother

As Julie read, Marti was aware of the reactions the others were having to it. Feelings were emerging in everyone, but rather than making a comment herself, or asking for input, she waited. It was important that Julie explore her feelings without their opinions influencing her. It was equally important that she and the others understand where Julie was coming from before making suggestions. So Marti proceeded carefully, walking Julie through the process that would allow her to see how this letter affected her. "Julie," she said, "your mother seems to have a totally different view of what happened that day. What is that like for you?"

It's too vast a question, Julie thought, physically shrinking into her chair even as she backed away from investigating further. Why did I bring this up? she asked herself. It's so embarrassing to have a mother like this. I wonder what everyone thinks of me now. But having brought it up, she couldn't erase the subject. So, she said, "This probably doesn't bother me as much as it does you. It's nothing new, you know. Having my mother blame me for everything is just a part of my life. That is, until I married Tom. Then, she had him to blame, too. What's interesting is that, somehow nothing is ever my brother's fault, even though he's had a serious drug and alcohol problem for years. But it's not his fault that he's incapable of holding a job for longer than a couple of months! My mom doesn't even see anything wrong with him sponging off her by living in her house and eating her food. And Eric is 34 years old!"

Compassionately, Marti asked, "How does it feel right now, as you're telling us about it?" Having already said the worst, Julie's answer came from the heart. "Awful," she said. "Everything about our relationship upsets me." Following up on that, Marti asked, "Upsets you? You're just upset?"

"Well," Julie conceded, hoping her chin wouldn't tremble. "I guess I'm angry, too. It's terrible when someone never sees your side of anything. It's like nothing I do is good enough and everything I do is wrong." Marti replied, "It must be hard not to get your mother's approval or attention in a positive way. How does that make you feel?" Then she gave Julie a chance to supply just the right description.

Now both tears and words flowed. "Unlovable," Julie said around the lump in her throat. Coming too, were the ghastly words: "Like I'm gross and disgusting. And it hurts, really hurts, to feel that way." Then, willing her tears to stop, she said, "I hate talking about it because it's so depressing!"

Marti was elated that Julie had provided five feeling words:

unlovable, gross, disgusting, hurt, and depressing. Not only was this indicative of Julie's growing recognition of her emotions, it also illustrated Julie's continuing trust in the Group. And it gave substantiation to something that Marti had been suspecting for some time – that Julie had been enduring unrecognized depression for a very long time. So Marti said, "While I can't say that your mother loves you, I can say that it's clear that she's needed you a lot. It's you she counts on to fix things for her. But things don't stay fixed for her. Instead, no matter what you do, she needs more and more all the time. It's your mother's inability to take responsibility for herself that has made you feel unlovable because she tells you that you are the source of her unhappiness. So there's nothing wrong with how you feel about her letter. Receiving it would upset, hurt, and sadden anyone. Besides, your mother is an adult. Solving her problems and making her happy is not your responsibility. What you did with your brother was the right thing to do. And so is keeping your limits and boundaries with your mother, although I know that it is quite trying!"

Julie, hanging on every encouraging word, said, "Intellectually, I know that what you're saying is true. But another part of me, probably my little girl, feels like I'm a defective daughter." Again, Marti pursued the feeling. "How does your little girl feel when she is expected to make life better?" Sighing, Julie said, "Like someone just ordered me to build a cathedral all by myself!" Paraphrasing, Marti said, "Sounds like your little girl feels overwhelmed and...."

Conscientiously, Julie finished the sentence. "Frightened," she replied. "Terrified, actually, because I don't know how to make things better." Leading her along, Marti asked, "What do you do when she feels that way?" Lightning-fast the answer returned. "I eat! Eating makes everything better."

Just as quickly, Marti asked, "How?"

"It takes the bad feelings away," Julie answered. "For a while, anyway. But afterward I hate myself!"

It's finally out in the open, thought Marti. To Julie, she said, "You've just identified a critical connection between feelings and food. When your little girl experiences things that make her uncomfortable, she eats for relief. But it's only temporary, and the feelings are never really gone. They've only been pushed down deep, deep inside. Over time, feelings that are covered up can lead to depression and that can sometimes make you want to eat even more. This creates a cycle that can't help but lead to weight gain." Surprised at how simple it sounded when it was said out loud, Julie said, "So if I take care of the depression I can lose weight?"

Marti said, "Depression could be a big part of your weight gain. Eating in response to feelings will lead to weight gain." Julie shook her head. Everything Marti said felt right, but she didn't know how to change it. So she asked, "What's the next step?" Marti turned to the others to ask, "How about the rest of you – any ideas?"

For some minutes Bobbie had been thinking how much easier it was to solve someone else's problems. Now, she suggested, "Using any language you want, write a return letter saying how you feel about what happened, and how you wish things could be different." When Julie gasped, Bobbie reassured her. "This letter is just for you, so you don't have to worry about hurting anyone's feelings." Julie looked at Marti to see what she thought. Marti nodded. "OK," Julie said. "I think I can do that."

"Later," Marti recommended, "you can write a more specific letter saying what upset you, what you want to change, and what kind of behavior you will tolerate from your mother. That's the one you will mail." Kate agreed, saying, "You need to do the same thing with your brother."

The thought of actually mailing anything threw Julie for a loop. "If my mother doesn't pay attention to what I say, she sure won't care what I write," she objected. "And unless he thinks there's a check inside, my brother won't even open the envelope." Here, Marti interjected, "What others do isn't important. The point is to find a way to get your feelings out. Writing them down is one way of doing that. It keeps you from having to stuff them inside." Not wanting to argue, Julie nodded. But she was thinking that while everything everyone said was true, they never had to deal with her family. It was time for someone else, and Bobbie volunteered.

Still reluctant to get caught up in feelings, Bobbie went back to the movement assignment. "You know," she said, "there were no classes in med school on nutrition or weight loss. Everyone just operated on the old belief that the solution to losing weight was simple, and they handed out the same old prescription: decrease calories and increase exercise! So when I read the assignment, I thought that this was the week you were going to validate that old standard. I told myself that if you were going to peddle the old carrot stick and jogging cure, I was just going to have to get used to being fat!" Marti mused, "You know, Bobbie, it sounds like you've reached a point where you can no longer go back to dieting. How does that feel?"

Cautious about giving too much of herself away, Bobbie said, "Kind of scary. There's nothing to fall back on if this doesn't work. This program is not easy; it's a lot of work. But if I don't do it, I know that nothing will ever change." Watching everyone agree with this assessment of what lay ahead, Marti knew that they were all in the same position of crossing the line of no return.

Then Bobbie changed subjects again. This time, it was about Garth. "I told you that he'd paid for all his charges," she said. "When he came home, he was carrying an expensive, new briefcase, and a bunch of packages he took right to his room. I couldn't help wondering how he could afford those things now, when he couldn't before. I guess he's not money-wise. I wonder if he thinks I'll always be there to bail him out. By the time I realized all of this, he was gone again. This time for three weeks." Kate, who had begun recognizing these behaviors when Bobbie first mentioned Garth's borrowing, wanted to tell her to boot the bastard out. Don't invest any more time in him, she wanted to say. But, she didn't.

It was just as well because Bobbie wasn't ready yet to hear a discouraging word about Garth even if true. Right now she was trying to decide whether she should bring up the fact that Garth had never contributed to the house payment. Not that he didn't do anything: he cooked for her when he was home and straightened the house and took out the garbage, but he didn't pay for anything. Just thinking about this made Bobbie feel disloyal. The truth was that she'd never asked him to help out financially. Now, feeling embarrassed as well as guilty, she decided to keep the housekeeping side of their relationship to herself. Instead, she switched subjects one more time. "My parents had their 35th wedding anniversary party," she said. "It was at the country club, of course; my mother wouldn't have it any other way. My sister and her husband were there, too." From her tone, the others could tell that the occasion left something to be desired.

"There I was in a room filled with beautiful, wealthy, perfect people," Bobbie continued. "But, despite my experience with other thoroughly boring evenings at the club, I'd decided to have a good time. I enjoyed myself even when my mother and sister gave those airy little gasps over my choice of entree. You should have heard them when I ordered dessert. You see," Bobbie explained, "because I love the raspberry chocolate cheesecake at the club, I intentionally saved room. If my mother and sister had bothered to look, they would have seen that I hadn't eaten everything on my plate." Here, Bobbie imitated their overly refined voices, "'Oh, none for me, thank you. I've eaten far too much already.' And they looked straight at me as they were saying it. Fortunately, my father and my brother-in-law followed with orders of their own. When dessert came and I took my first bite, Mom gave this enormous sigh and whispered to my sister loud enough for me to hear, 'It's okay, Melanie. Bobbie's figure isn't as important to her as ours are to us.' But," Bobbie said, "I didn't let it bother me. I ate every last morsel and it was wonderful. Now I'll admit to you that I didn't eat it because I was hungry, but it was one of those times that I'd have devoured tin cans just to annoy my mother. And it did, but I got my comeuppance later, when we went out to get our cars."

Her joy in having triumphed quickly disappearing, Bobbie said, "I'd parked my van myself because it's faster than valet service. My parents and everyone else were still waiting for their cars when I drove by. Dad waved, but Mom turned away as if she didn't know me. I felt really bad about embarrassing her. But it could have been worse I hadn't had time to clean out my car. It would have been my luck to have the valet open my door and have all my stuff fall out. It's really disgusting; I don't even know what's in there. But it made me realize that I really do want to have time to take care of the things in my life. I don't like having my car full of junk, so I ignore it. Like I ignore my unfurnished house."

Bobbie had told far more than she'd intended, and it exhausted her. Seeing this, Marti said, "Speaking of the dinner, I'm really proud of you for not allowing anyone else to influence your order. That showed that you really believe yourself to be the best judge of what your body needs and wants. I'm proud, too, of how you handled what we call 'the diet police.' The diet police, like your mother, decide what you shouldn't eat based upon your body size. They tell you when to diet, and how. It's a real milestone when you realize that the diet police have no power unless you give it to them." Revived somewhat by the praise, Bobbie said, "That's true! But those people know better than anyone how to make you feel bad!"

"It sounds like it felt good to rebel," said Marti. "How did your body feel afterward?"

Bobbie remembered all too well how she felt. "I love bernaise sauce, but it was too rich, and the cheesecake was just too much. By the time I got home, my stomach was unsettled. But that was just as well, too, because for the first time I realized that my body doesn't feel good when I eat that much rich food. So this week, I've been trying to be more aware of the difference between being satisfied instead of full or stuffed."

Thrilled, Marti said, "Good work!" Bobbie smiled, glad that she'd told them about the party instead of giving them the full story on Garth. Then it was time for Emily.

"It's been a bad week for me," she said. "I didn't have time to work on the assignment because, along with everything else, my parents called to say they were coming home." Earnestly, she said, "I'm beginning to see things about my parents that relate to my weight." Then, her eyes showing just a hint of tears, she paused, gulped, and said, "I'm still so upset about what happened that I don't think I can talk about it without crying. So," she said without the laugh they'd come to expect, "I'm apologizing early!"

Going on to say that her parents had been away for a month, visiting relatives, she'd decided that it would be a nice welcome home to get the whole family together. "Except by the time last Sunday rolled around, I didn't have the energy to cook a lot of food, so I did something I'd never done before I bought deli food." The reaction to this went from surprise to admiration. "It was a scary decision," Emily admitted. "But I've been so tired lately that I decided that if I cooked, I'd be too exhausted to enjoy the party." Kate, who couldn't agree more, said, "That was a smart decision!"

Giving a small smile acknowledging the praise, Emily said, "I ordered the same amount of food I would normally cook and decorated the table with a 'Welcome Home' sign my daughter made. It looked really nice, but when Mom arrived, the first thing she said was, 'Isn't this too much food?' Then she went into her usual lecture on 'waste not, want not.'"

Kate was the first to react, curious to know if the rest of the family had objected to this rudeness. Emily replied that they hadn't because it was nothing unusual. "But it did put a damper on things," she said, "especially when Mom made it a point to complain about not being able to eat the lasagne or roast beef that I usually fix for these events. It's true that the food wasn't as good as mine, but I had more fun because I wasn't so tired."

"And," she said, "this was the first time that my parents had ever seen me eat the same food as everyone else." What? Even Marti was surprised. So Emily explained, "I've never before eaten regular food in front of my parents." Now Emily elaborated. "I've told you before that my mother fixed 'special' food for me, and I was never allowed to have birthday cake, but it was even worse than that. My mother wasn't mean about it she was so worried about me being fat that she went to all this extra trouble. It's just that being singled out that way made me feel defective. Especially when she prefaced each meal with 'This is Emily's special food because she wants to lose weight, don't you, Emily?' So you can imagine her reaction when I didn't bring out my usual diet food but went though the buffet instead. I didn't dare look at her while I was choosing what I wanted to eat and how much. But then and this is where things started getting really weird before I got a chance to sit down and eat, one of the kids asked me to fix a glitch on the video tape. When I came back to where I thought I'd left my plate, it was gone. I couldn't find it anywhere. So I gave up and went through the line a second time. Just as I finished fixing my plate, my neighbor called to say that our dog was out. I put my plate on the kitchen counter and went out to get him. And when I came back, guess what – it was gone. Again!"

During this last part of Emily's story, Kate started narrowing her eyes. Julie's hand had flown to her mouth and her eyes had grown wider with each word. Now, Margaret began shaking her head, whispering, "No! She wouldn't!"

Emily leaned forward, saying, "Then I knew something was going on. So I filled a third plate, put it on the sideboard, and went through the kitchen and into the hall, just as if I was going to the bathroom. Only, I turned around just in time to see my mother rush into the kitchen with my plate. Even though I had my suspicions, I honestly couldn't believe it when I saw her scraping all that food into the trash compactor. I mean," Emily said, her voice indignant, "talk about waste!"

"Did she see you?" Margaret asked.

"No. And something inside forced me to speak up, to ask what she thought she was doing."

"What did she say?" Julie asked.

"She didn't say anything. She was startled, but it didn't stop her, she continuing doing what she was doing. Now," Emily asked everyone, "wouldn't you be embarrassed if you were caught doing something like that? My mom wasn't in the slightest! So I said, 'Mom, that's my food and so were the other two plates that you threw away!' And she said, 'Well, honey, this kind of food isn't good for you.'"

"You know," Emily confided, "that brought back memories of every other time she's said that. But when I tried to tell her that it wasn't up to her to make that decision, she pooh-poohed me."

"Did you put up with that?" demanded Kate.

"No, and I think it was because I was so hungry," Emily replied. "I told her that I hadn't eaten all day! That's when she said that I must have something in the house that was good for me and went to my freezer. That's where I lost it," Emily said. Her voice growing stronger, she reported, "I said, 'Stay out of my freezer. I know exactly what I want to eat and it's out on the buffet table.'" Then I went back and fixed a fourth plate and ate every bit of it. But, while it felt good, by that time I'd really lost my appetite because I was upset. And scared. It's the first time I ever talked that way to my mom. Here I am, all grown up everywhere else, but not when my mom and dad are around."

For a few moments, no one could think of anything to say. Emily's situation was far worse than any of them could have imagined. Margaret, who'd never had anyone openly restrict her food, was trying to understand what Emily's mother was thinking. All of them knew that Emily had handled the situation better than they would have. But Marti was the one who said it aloud. "Emily, you did a great job, and it took a lot of courage to confront your mother like that." Then, to the entire Group, she said, "Emily's example underscores what you've been learning for the past 13 weeks: NO ONE has the right to tell you what to eat!" Emily, although she was still angry at the encounter, blossomed with this tribute. It felt good to have everyone understand how difficult it had been. Yet she wasn't finished with her bad news. "The awful thing is that my parents ended up staying with us. They'll be with us for the next few weeks because they're having work done on their house. After only four days, how I feed my family and myself is already turning into a battle. So you can see," she went on, "with my mother mentally measuring and counting everything I put on the table, I don't know if I can handle it."

Right away, Kate asked, "Don't you have brothers and sisters here in town? Couldn't your parents stay with them?" Emily admitted that this was so, but her parents preferred to stay with her for some reason.

Listening to this, each of them knew what Emily was going through. In the past it had been easier to give in than to argue, especially with a parent. No matter how adult you were away from your parents, there were tones of voice and phrases that could return you to childhood in a flash. So, Marti thought, Emily might be afraid that with her parents moving in, she might lose her adult status. Marti addressed that by saying, "It's difficult to be around people who feel that their job in life is to control your every move, particularly around food. How does that make you feel?" "Like there must be something wrong with me," Emily admitted, her eyes awash. "Actually," she said, "I've always felt that being fat made me feel less than human." A quizzical look from Marti encouraged her to continue. Even more softly, she replied, "My weight has always been the focus of my mother's attention – like it was her duty in life to make me thin."

"What would be different if you were thin?" asked Marti.

"I guess I could finally be part of the family," Emily whispered.

This was an extremely emotional moment. Everyone identified with what Emily was feeling. This, they recognized, was part of a core issue they all shared. On one level or another, each of them knew what it felt like to be an outsider in their own families. The pain of acknowledging that brought tears to every eye. "Sounds like," Marti said, "you are letting out a lot of feelings that you have held silent for a long time. What was it like for you to say them out loud?"

Wiping the tears away, Emily replied, "I've never said this to anyone else, and it's embarrassing to say what happened to me." Looking up at the Group, she continued, "But it feels good to get it out in the open – kind of a relief."

"I'm proud of you, Emily," Marti said, "for revealing what your mother has always done to you with food. It had to be uncomfortable for you to look at that. Now, I have a question: if you had kept it all inside, would this have been one of those times you would have turned to food?" Emily took a minute to consider this. Then, with a sigh, she said, "Yes!" So Marti asked, "Have you seen any changes in your food since they've been with you?"

Biting her lip, Emily said, "I noticed that I started feeling hungry the day they moved in and, now, I'm constantly thinking about food, again. I'm afraid that in the next three weeks I'm going to lose everything I've learned here."

Marti nodded. "It's like all those old fears of not having enough to eat are coming back," she said. "Sounds like you need ways to stay centered on remaining aware of your needs and taking care of them in the next few weeks. How about the rest of you? Any ideas?"

Julie had one. "You could take some time every day just for yourself." Kate suggested. "If you need to talk, call me; I'm either at work, or at home."

And Margaret volunteered, "You can call me, too."

"And it's okay to do things without your parents," Marti recommended. "It would be good for you and your family to occasionally have a meal together away from them. You will know when you need to do this. Something else that will be extremely helpful is to journal." Picking up her notebook, Marti pointed to the page on the right and said, "This page is titled 'Journal'. Part of it is devoted to your weekly assignment questions, but there's plenty of room left for you to write about anything that is bothering you. It would be helpful for all of you to do this: journaling teaches you to observe what's going on in your life. Writing down whatever comes to mind helps you to see problems more objectively. Then you can more readily see the choices you have to resolve them. It also gives you a place to unload your concerns so that you don't have to stuff them inside."

"Thank you," Emily said, and everyone was pleased to see that she looked far more hopeful than she had at the beginning. "Everything you've said really helps. Thank you." And, although Kate had been dreading this moment, it was her turn. She began with an apology.

"I'm sorry for not being here the last few weeks," she said. "I left town unexpectedly because Ed started in on one of his benders again. I just couldn't take his drinking anymore." Every night, she told them, he'd come home late, angry and full of accusations. When he couldn't get a rise out of her, he drank himself into oblivion. If it had been limited to home, she might have been able to stand it, but he had become hostile at work, too. He'd begun calling her names in front of employees, and one day he threw his coffee cup at her and that was it!

"I went to Reno to visit one son," she said, "then to Seattle to see the other. I told myself, 'Let's see how well Ed runs the company without me!'"

"Did he know where you were?" asked Bobbie, marveling at Kate's courage in walking away from everything.

"I gave him a dose of his own medicine. I left without a word,"

Kate said, with some satisfaction. "The employees knew where I was, so they could phone me if they needed, but as far as Ed knew, I'd disappeared off the face of the earth." Not surprisingly, when she came home, she'd found problems everywhere, with everyone and Ed had disappeared, too. "I'd worried a lot about the business while I was gone because Ed hadn't been at work enough to know what was going on. I'm afraid," she said, "if he doesn't shape up, we're going to lose the business." With this out in the open, Marti wanted her to take a closer look inward. So she asked, "What was going on inside that forced you to leave?"

Even after all these weeks in the program, Marti's interest in what took place inside of her took Kate by surprise. Suddenly, she felt vulnerable. "When Ed started drinking again, and then started throwing things at me, I was afraid of what was going to happen if I stuck around. I had to get away – it wasn't safe anymore."

"What would have happened?" asked Margaret.

"The more he drinks, the uglier he gets – and I got tired of hearing how awful I am. I left because I couldn't stand being around his vile mouth and terrible temper." But Marti still wanted to know about what happened to Kate when Ed behaved this way. "So you could see him becoming more and more belligerent – and verbally attacking you. What is it like for you to be around him when he's like that?"

"There's a part of me that used to believe that he was right – that somehow, I'd messed up again. So the only thing I could do was to try not to cause any more problems so I'd stand there and take it. I'm no longer so naive. This last time, I knew that he was wrong to talk to me that way. Still, I feel totally helpless when he's drunk and out of control. There's a look that he has that scares me half to death. Three weeks ago when I saw it in his eyes, I knew something bad was going to happen, and it was time to get away."

Marti pressed on. "I wonder what you were feeling at the moment you decided to leave?" Kate had the perfect word: "Cornered. And I didn't dare let him see how scared I was." From the tone in her voice, Marti could hear that Kate was a little embarrassed about this admission. Reassuringly, Marti said, "You did the right thing. But it wasn't 'running away,' it was protecting yourself."

Kate struggled with that concept. "I keep wondering if I should have stayed, but I was so scared. I guess that shows how weak I am. A strong person wouldn't have those feelings!" Quickly, Marti asked, "So you believe that only weak people have feelings? And if you don't have feelings, then you must be strong!"

"That's right," said Kate, although she found no comfort in saying it. The others, newly in touch with their own feelings, were extremely interested in what Marti would have to say about this.

"Having feelings," Marti said, "is an essential part of being human. It has nothing to do with anyone's strength or weakness. In fact, feelings give us direction, telling us where our limits and boundaries are, give us a way to bond with others and to know when danger is present. Without feelings, we cannot be fully protected. It would be like being blind without a white cane. But, somewhere, you got the message that feelings are bad." While Kate was assimilating this, Marti was thinking that, for Kate, running was one of her ways of dealing with her feelings: first she ran from Ed – could she have been running from Group, too? So Marti said, "The last time you were here, you told us about Ed and that brought up a lot of feelings. What was it like for you?"

"Dangerous!" Kate said. "I was expecting someone to tell me that I was a wimp that I should just stop sniveling about things and get a divorce."

So, thought Marti, that was it. Kate was afraid of being forced into something she wasn't ready to do. So Marti acknowledged Kate for her courage by saying, "It must have been hard to come tonight." Kate sighed, grateful for the understanding. "Yes, it was," she said. Marti, feeling that it was important for Kate to clarify further, asked, "Do you think that not coming to class last week had something to do with having been so open about your feelings the last time you were here?" Kate was very clear about that. "Partly." she said. "I'd been forced to look at things that I'd been avoiding for a long time. And then after this last incident, I was too ashamed to come back." Whispering, now, she added, "I didn't know what you all would think of me."

Seeing how exposed Kate was, Marti asked, "Now that you're here and talking with us, what is it like?" Still whispering, Kate replied, "Amazing. All of you listened and didn't criticize me."

"You are the best judge of what is right for you," said Marti. "We're here to support you in any decisions that you make." Then, bringing the discussion around to the reason they were all there, Marti spoke to everyone, "In the past, we've all used food to deal with our problems and feelings. Now that we're not doing that anymore, all those emotions that we thought were dead and buried are surfacing again. When we use food to take care of feelings, it allows us to deny what's really causing the pain and nothing gets resolved. Everything stays the same except your weight. So, Kate, what happened with your food in the last three weeks?"

Kate had been nodding her head in agreement as Marti spoke. "Well," she said, "I've gone back to snacking late at night." Marti said, "With all the feelings that you've experienced in the last few weeks, it makes sense that you would return to your old ways of coping. You've done a very good job of letting yourself feel your feelings. Now, do you think there's a relationship between Ed and your unconscious eating late at night?"

For an instant, all Kate heard was a voice deep inside of herself saying, "Divorce him, divorce him, divorce him!" Terrified, she said, "I don't know; I'd better think about that for a while." Glancing at her watch, she was relieved that her 15 minutes were up. Good, there was no more time for questions. Or answers.

Marti handed out the next week's assignment and everyone said their goodbyes. But when she, too, left the office a few minutes later,

Kate was waiting for her. "Can I make an appointment with you?" she asked. Marti smiled. "Sounds like a good idea," Marti said. "There isn't much time in class to work on everything." So they checked their schedules and made an appointment. Crossing the parking lot, Marti thought about Kate. This request for help really reflected the growth Kate had made since starting Group. It was a big risk, Marti knew, for Kate to be willing to look even deeper into herself.

CHAPTER SEVEN

Where's My Money?

Week Fifteen: The Connection Between Money & Weight

*L*OOKING OVER HER NOTES before the women arrived, Marti was thinking that there were an infinite number of ways to feel hungry. It wasn't exclusively limited to food. The hard part was that for most of these women, food was the only solution to any and all feelings of deprivation. All of them were still surprised when she brought up other seemingly unrelated things in their lives. It was, Marti knew, the remaining vestige of their old diet thinking; the belief that if you wanted to lose weight, the only things you ever discussed were food, inches, and pounds. Every week, their awareness of other hungers was growing, but their latest assignments – connecting time, money, and organization of space to eating unconsciously – was still a stretch. Of course, every day brought them closer, so as Marti went down the hall to the waiting room, she smiled. What, she wondered, had the women discovered this past week?

As the women entered, they continued their chatter about conversations begun in the parking lot and reception room. Only

Emily, Marti noted, seemed less sociable than usual. The first to take her chair, she made no effort to be a part of the busy bustle that always accompanied the first few minutes of opening their books and removing their pens. Marti started the evening with, "For the past few weeks we've been trying to identify all the other hungers you may be experiencing, and how they might be connected to food."

Everyone but Emily smiled and exchanged glances. Had they ever! But Marti was asking, "Since we have a lot of ground to cover tonight, why don't we get started – who wants to be first?"

"I will," Bobbie said, energetically. Everyone's attention was drawn by Bobbie's surprising eagerness to share. "You know, it wasn't until I did the assignment that I realized just how much money I'm spending. I thought that because my checkbook balanced each month and I was able to pay my bills, everything was under control. Frankly, it's always been hard to find time at the end of the month to pay bills. So the thought never occurred to me to sit down and figure out where my money was going." Seeing frowns on everyone's faces, Bobbie continued before anyone could say anything. Putting her hands up as if to block their questions, she said, "I know, I know: time is not an excuse anymore. I have to take time to do these things, which is what I did this past weekend." Now, everyone understood Bobbie's enthusiasm. "That's great! said Margaret. "I'm proud of you," smiled Marti. It struck Bobbie how silly this was. It's embarrassing, she remarked to herself, that a grown woman like me is getting praise for doing something I should have been doing all along. But it felt good to get congratulated for it, anyway. She went on with her story.

"Saturday morning, I had this great idea of reading the paper in bed for once. Then I saw it – a furniture sale, and in the store's ad I saw exactly what I wanted for my bedroom. I was so excited that I got up, got dressed, and went to the ATM to transfer money from my savings to my checking account. That's when I found out that I didn't have enough money in the account. That really confused me because I know how much I've been putting in savings the past few months. But there wasn't as much as I thought there should be. I couldn't stop thinking about it – where had the money gone? So when I got home, I went through the last three month's worth of bank statements, and found that I'd withdrawn a lot more money than I'd thought."

Her enthusiasm diminishing fast, Bobbie went on to explain, "You see, I haven't kept tabs on how much I take out. It's that damned ATM in the hospital that makes it so easy." Interesting, Marti was thinking, Bobbie is as unconscious about her money as she was with her food. But Bobbie was continuing.

"It's not all my fault – there have been a couple of times in the last few months when Garth has run short of cash, for things like car insurance. So I loaned him the money. The bad thing about that is there's a lot more money that I can't account for. On top of it, I realized that Garth has never paid me back for the money he's borrowed." Everyone was shocked. "I hate to think, Bobbie said, "how much money he's borrowed in the three years we've been living together." Margaret was having a hard time understanding this. "Doesn't he feel guilty taking your money and not paying you back?" she asked.

Fearing condemnation of Garth, Bobbie came to his defense. "He can't be blamed for the whole thing," she said. "I spent some of that money, too. Besides, it's not like he's a bad person, or anything. He comes from one of those old, established families that has trust funds for their heirs. But it's hard to borrow from them, especially when you're in a hurry. Then there's his work. He's really good at what he does, but with his clients, he likes to wine and dine them at the finest places. Not only is that expensive, but that kind of entertaining also requires that he has to have the right clothes and car. His company reimburses him, but I'm sure that his budget doesn't cover what Garth spends."

Knowing that it was important for Bobbie to investigate this issue a little more closely, Marti decided to comment directly with, "So, Bobbie, what you're saying is that when Garth gets into a bind, you feel the need to help him. He forgets to pay you back, and you forget that you've loaned it to him! Then, when you want money for something that's important to you, it's not there. It's as if your money is more for Garth than for yourself."

What Marti said made Bobbie very uncomfortable, not only because she suspected it was true, but also because she anticipated a forthcoming question that was not going to be easy to answer. She was right, for Marti said, "I wonder if the way you handle money has anything to do with the way your parents handled their money."

Bobbie took a moment to focus, then said, "My father handled the money. Mother spent far more money than Dad wanted in order to maintain the family's social standing. That meant the best of everything for herself, the house, Melanie, and me. It never mattered to Dad if we had the best or not. Anyway, he was born into a country club family and my mother wasn't. I can remember my parents having arguments about Mom's spending. We could hear them yelling in their bedroom, and Dad shouting, 'No more! This is your budget, and you have to make do with what we have.' Then he would warn her that he'd take away the checkbook and credit cards if she didn't stop spending so much. My sister and I figured out that Mother always went shopping after their fights to get back at him for being so tight. When he found out, he'd give her the silent treatment. They never solved the problem, they just kept fighting. I hated it. There were times I thought they would end up in divorce!" There, Bobbie stopped.

Taking advantage of the pause, Marti interpreted what Bobbie had said. "It sounds like your father would go along until he reached a point of feeling totally out of control with your mother's spending. To regain control, he'd establish verbal limits. What he didn't realize is that his limits took away your mother's only way of feeling important and powerful. She hated that, and fought back the only way she knew how. It's as if the money made your mother feel more desirable to others. Without it, she was ordinary, and believed that no one would want to be around her. In your family, whoever had the money had the power and control. So the fights may not have been just about money!"

For Bobbie, Marti's statements were profound. Looking up, she caught the therapist's smile and said, "That's exactly right. Nothing could be more important to my mother than getting her way."

"Do you see anything similar in the way you deal with money?" asked Marti. Her thoughts racing, Bobbie was not sure. "Garth and I never talk about money," she said. "Neither one of us knows what's going on with our own money, or each other's." Taking a deep breath, she continued, with, "Maybe I don't want to discuss it because it might end up in an argument. I guess I feel like I've reached the same point that my father always did – that I have to do something to stop our runaway spending. So I need to talk to Garth. But I don't know what I'll do if we fight about it," she worried. Having identified what was wrong and what had to be done, Bobbie was apprehensive. Her worst fears were that she'd end up like her parents.

Marti, wanting to push Bobbie a little more, asked, "Here's a hypothetical question: What would happen if Garth had an endless supply of money?" Bobbie was quick to answer. "I guess he wouldn't need me any more."

"And what do you think he'd do if he didn't need you?" asked Marti.

"He would have no reason to stay – so I guess he'd leave." Saying it out loud gave Bobbie a sinking feeling in the pit of her stomach. Marti continued. "So, are you saying that by giving him money when he needs it, he has a reason to stay in the relationship?"

Bobbie squirmed in her seat, challenged beyond her comfort zone and hoping she would be finished soon. Finally, she spoke. "I used to think that by helping Garth I was showing him how much I cared."

What struck Marti was that a woman with such intelligence and compassion for others couldn't see the value in herself as a person. So she said, "It is so sad that you believe that Garth would find no other reason to be with you except for your money," said Marti. "Where did that belief come from?"

Bobbie knew right away. "You've already answered that: my mother," she said. "She showed me that money makes you desirable and special. Without it, you're nothing." Smiling, Marti said, "Is it possible that your father also contributed to this belief?" Seeing Bobbie hesitate, she expanded her point. "He punished your mother with silence, but never followed through with his threats. Maybe he felt that his money was the only reason your mother stayed with him. In other words, it was his only value!" Bobbie nodded. "Your mother and father could be more alike than you think."

"That never occurred to me," Bobbie replied. "But now that you mention it..." Her eyebrows rose in contemplation. What Marti said had connected, and everyone could see it written on her face. At this point, Marti decided against pushing further. This was, after all, not individual therapy. So she changed the focus by asking, "How do feelings of deprivation fit into all of this?"

The shift caught Bobbie by surprise. Thinking it over, she answered, "The way things are now, I don't have money for the things I want. It didn't matter so much before, but now I can see that I've gone without: look at my car. No, look at my house," she exclaimed. "No wonder I eat so much!"

"That's great," congratulated Marti. "You've just identified another hunger – a big one! When you don't have the money you want and need, you feel deprived, you turn to food, and you gain weight. How could you handle your money differently so you won't have to go without?"

Almost as if she was thinking aloud, or practicing this new

thought, Bobbie said, "I need to be more aware of what I'm doing with my money. And, if Garth – or anybody – asks me for a loan, I have to decide whether I can afford it or not. If not, I need to say no." Only Bobbie knew how hard this was going to be. Mainly because she and Garth never had time to talk. So if she came at him with something this decisive, she feared she would be jeopardizing their relationship. What would she do if he refused? How would she feel if he left? Oh God, she thought, what would my mother say? Caught up in her own thoughts, Bobbie suddenly realized that her time was up, and she said that someone could go next.

Julie raised her hand. "First, I'd like to report that the garage is finished and we can actually get two cars in there. It's so nice; everything is put away and there is so much room. Tom is thrilled!" Julie took a minute to look around the table. Then, gathering courage, she said, "I finally wrote a letter to my mom, but I haven't mailed it. Then, last Tuesday when I got home from work there was another message on my answering machine. I almost died when I heard her voice saying, 'Not that you care, but your brother's disappeared again.' Then she hung up. This isn't," Julie reassured everyone, "anything new. Eric is always taking off and it always sends Mom into a panic. What is different is that I didn't drop everything to look for him. Why should I?" she asked. "No matter how it turns out, my mother would find a way to make it all my fault, anyway. So, I'm glad that I wrote that letter because it reminds me that my brother isn't my responsibility. I decided that I'm not going to call her back. I am worried about him, but I realize that I can't keep trying to rescue him when he doesn't want to be saved. Still, I can't help feeling like a bad sister and a worse daughter."

Right away, Marti reinforced what Julie had done. "Good job, Julie; you are right to establish that boundary with your mother and brother." Raising a wan smile, Julie said, "I really needed to hear that." Marti smiled reassuringly, while everyone else was thinking that Julie – the most quiet and withdrawn of them all – had come a long way to be able to stand up to her mother. Smiling back, Julie went on to report what she'd discovered about her finances.

"I have to laugh because I thought this assignment was going to be easy. So I felt kind of stupid when I couldn't answer most of questions because I haven't the faintest idea what Tom does with our money. Every payday, all I do is hand my paycheck over to him. He handles everything."

"Is that arrangement all right with you?" asked Marti.

"Well, he's really good at it. Except something came up this week that I couldn't believe." Julie went on to explain that she had a friend who was getting married in a couple of weeks. "I wanted to get a new dress, so I went shopping. I found exactly what I wanted, but then I felt so silly – standing there wondering if I ought to ask my husband whether I should write a check or use the charge card. I went ahead and charged it, even though it was more than I usually spend. Actually, it was a lot more than I usually spend. I was really nervous what Tom would say when he found out, and couldn't decide whether I'd tell him right away or later. So I took it home and hid it in the closet, figuring I'd tell him when the time was right." From the chuckles around the table, Julie suspected that, maybe, the others had done the same thing at one time or another. "The thing is," Julie said, "I didn't know when the bill was coming. So I had to tell him what I'd done sooner than I thought. You know what? The credit card company had already called him to verify the expense the day I bought it. He already knew what I'd spent." Her expression was one of such amazement that everyone had to laugh. "He didn't tell me to take it back or anything," Julie added, "Instead, he smiled. I couldn't believe he wasn't mad at me for spending so much money on a dress, but he shook his head and said that we could afford it." To herself, Julie thought that she'd hungered to hear him say that he was glad because she deserved it. But he'd just turned back to his computer.

Right away, Marti recognized that in giving total responsibility to her husband, Julie had made herself an unequal partner. Wanting to investigate Julie's feelings about this, Marti said, "It must be difficult to want something and not know if you can afford it. Not only that, but that you wondered if you needed permission to buy it."

"It's always been hard for me to ask for anything, whether I needed it or not!" Julie said.

"Always?" asked Marti.

Julie nodded. "I don't remember a whole lot before Dad left. But I do remember that everything changed after the divorce. We didn't have much, so I usually didn't get the things I wanted," she explained. "I guess my most vivid memory is Grandmother's favorite answer whenever I asked for something: 'You can't have everything you want in this life!' As a teenager, I always encountered a scene whenever I asked for something because Mom always told me I expected too much. She told me how selfish I was to want things when I knew her financial situation."

Emily remarked, "No wonder you have a hard time asking for things." Bobbie asked, "Does your husband expect you to justify all your spending?" Julie denied this, but had to add, "but maybe that's because most of my purchases are for everyone else. I almost never buy anything for me. Besides, I don't know what we can afford."

"Does that ever lead to not buying the things you really need or want?" asked Marti. Wondering if Marti was going to suggest that she take over doing the bills periodically, Julie said, "Yes, but not knowing is worth it as long as I don't have to make out the checks and balance the checkbook; I've got too much to do as it is!" The last was stated adamantly enough to surprise Marti. Hmm, she thought, that's an interesting aside. Julie needed to explore that. So Marti asked, "What feelings came up when you knew you wanted the dress but were afraid that you didn't have enough money – and might not be able to have it?"

Julie found the answer to that a struggle. So she fended it off with, "I'm used to going without things that I really want."

"Well," Marti said, coming at the question from another angle. "If the dress was food – something you really wanted to eat – how would you feel if you were afraid you couldn't have it?"

That was easy, and Julie said, "Robbed. Cheated… Deprived!"

"Mmmmn hmm!" said Marti. "Is it possible that the same feeling might come up when you face having to go without other things you want?" Julie searched that question inside. On the surface, equating a dress with food seemed ridiculous. But when you really looked at it, what Marti asked was true. "Now that you mention it," Julie replied, "it feels the same."

"So what do you do with that feeling of going without?" Marti asked. Mystified, Julie replied with a question: "What do I do with it?" Around the table, the others got it. Eat, they thought, sending the word toward her telepathically. Julie said, "I guess the right answer would be that I eat." Knowing that Julie wasn't owning it yet, Marti said, "If that's the case, do you find that eating solves the problem?" Marti gave Julie a little time, but didn't let up even when Julie said, "I don't know." Feeling that Julie needed some help, Marti suggested a possibility. "If your husband is handling all of your financial affairs, it puts you at a disadvantage – and that can make you feel like an unequal partner. So, the problem here may be that in not knowing how much money is available, you choose to go without – which leads to deprivation, which leads to eating. What could you do to make this better for you?"

It showed on Julie's face that she didn't like where the conversation was going; she found out long ago that knowing a little made you responsible for a lot. "I could find out more about our financial situation," she admitted. "But I hate handling money and paying bills!"

"A lot of people don't like doing that," Marti said. "But you can know what your finances are without assuming responsibility for writing checks and balancing bank statements." Now, that had never occurred to Julie before. Seeing this on her face, Marti waited for her to absorb the provocative new thought. For Julie, it was an entirely new approach to money. Knowing that she would need time to assimilate this, Marti finished with, "Both you and Tom work hard. Maybe it would help to have a plan that reserved a certain amount of money each month for each of you to spend any way you want. It's a good idea to decide together on an upper limit at which you will check with the other to make sure that it's okay. Everyone needs to realize that asking is not a matter of getting permission. Rather, it's consideration because whenever you spend more than the plan allows, it may take away money allocated for something else – and that has to be through mutual agreement." Hearing this, Julie went quiet again. She'd never considered the old money arrangement a problem. Now, it definitely felt like one. The question in her mind was, how long had she been eating over this? Then, what will Tom say when I tell him? Her attention came back to the room when she realized that the others were still waiting and she said, "It never occurred to me that I would feel this way about finances. I just thought our way was the way it should be." Smiling at the others, she signaled that she was through.

Emily picked up from there. "Our finances are fine: I handle everything, which is fine with me because it's just an extension of my job. Besides, my husband has no interest in money." Hmmmm, Marti wondered. After fifteen years of marriage, is Emily still satisfied with that arrangement, or had it become too heavy a burden? Does this cause any problem between Emily and her husband? And how does her being tired all the time fit into it? Most likely, Marti surmised, her fatigue could come from the feeling that she had to do everything. So when it's time to do anything for herself, she has no energy left to do it, which makes her feel deprived. Emily interrupted Marti's thoughts with, "One thing I did realize this week is that I really hate my job."

What a bombshell! No one had ever suspected that Emily wasn't happy with her work. Going on in a very weary voice, Emily said, "The work never ends, so I don't have the satisfaction of finishing anything. What's worse is that I'm not getting paid enough for the amount of work that I do, or for the responsibilities that I have. When I said something to Dave, he suggested that I ask for a raise. I did… they gave it to me… and I still hate my job."

Julie, who loved hers, asked, "What are you going to do?" Emily replied, "I'm actually thinking about going back to school." Another bombshell! With everything Emily had to do, how was she going to carry all those classes and do all that homework?

Obviously Emily had given this a lot of thought because she had a ready answer. "I quit when I got pregnant because working full-time, going to school, and caring for a baby would be too much. But it didn't matter then, I was thrilled to death to be pregnant." Then, with more enthusiasm than she'd shown in a long time, Emily said, "But, now, I think I want to be a lawyer." Margaret thought this was a great idea. "You'd be a wonderful attorney!" she enthused. "With your intelligence and work ethic, you can't help but be successful!" Before Marti could say anything, Julie was saying, "Wow! You sure are brave to leave a well-paying job in the hope of being happy somewhere else." Emily hardly acknowledged Julie's caution, going on with, "Dave says we can afford to do this if it's what I want," she said. "How the kids will take this, however, is going to be interesting. It's really going to cut down on the amount of money and things they're used to getting. But I'm ready for that," she said, "I guess the thing I'm really worried about is not doing my share to support the family."

Knowing how big an issue this can be to some women, Marti asked, "What is it about Dave carrying the load that makes you uncomfortable?" Thinking for a moment, Emily said, "Since this will be a new experience, I'm not sure how it's going to work, but I know I'll be giving up having my own money, and the family is going to have to make sacrifices, too. And," here she hesitated before going on, "what if I go back to school and fail?"

Addressing potential failure, Marti said, "Changing a profession is a big risk – and failure is a part of that risk. But, so is success! Failures are a part of life, and we learn a lot about ourselves from them. Besides, you cannot have happiness without taking risks." Marti went on to praise Emily. "I am really impressed that you were able to come to these revelations with your parents around."

Emily sighed. "It's been a real eye-opener being in constant contact with them. I'd be lying if I didn't admit that they're driving me nuts. You can't believe how domineering and rigid these people are. For them, a menu is non-negotiable: they have always had a specific meal for every night of the week." Seeing Margaret frown, Emily explained. "In my mother's house, dinner is determined by the day of the week. Monday is always spaghetti night, Tuesday is meatloaf. Even for lunch, my parents still eat exactly the same things: half a peanut butter sandwich each, two thirds of a glass of milk, a piece of seasonal fruit or two fig newtons. For them, leftovers are the Devil's handiwork. Well, I don't live that way! I cook more than enough because I want to make sure no one goes hungry."

"I like your way better than theirs," Kate chuckled. Managing a small smile, Emily said, "They make all sorts of comments about me wasting food. So, one night, Mom insisted upon cooking dinner – to show me how it was supposed to be done. She fixed fried chicken because it was Wednesday. Just like when I was growing up, Mom prepared all of the plates in the kitchen, so each serving was carefully measured: two pieces of chicken for my father and Dave, one piece each for the rest of us. If you can believe, she managed to make one can of green beans serve six people. Actually, there was also one tiny baked potato apiece. And that's it! When my son and daughter asked for more chicken, my mother told them that she thought they'd had enough – and it was close to bedtime anyway. I just wish that you could have seen the expression on their faces! I felt so bad that I lied and told my mother that we had an errand to run for school. Then the four of us escaped to a nearby restaurant to finish our dinner." Rubbing her temples with her fingers, Emily said,

"And that's when it came to me: Mom's always controlled everyone's food. I thought I was the only one who couldn't have an extra portion, but that's not true – no one could because she never made enough for second helpings. It's like I said, to my parents, leftovers are the Devil's handiwork." Now everyone could see that this long recital had taken its toll, for Emily sighed again.

Everyone had opinions on this, and they weren't a bit backward about sharing them. When they'd finished venting their outrage, Marti said, "It's good that you saw that you were not the only one being deprived and controlled. Growing up in this restrictive atmosphere around food and money may have influenced some of your adult behaviors and attitudes, I wonder how you view the concept of enough."

Emily replied, "That's easy – there was never enough – you made do with what was given to you. It didn't matter what you wanted or thought you needed – you didn't get it!" Marti asked a question that brought Emily straight up in her chair. "Do you suppose that there is a connection between having enough, fearing the loss of your own personal money, and needing to control your family's budget?"

Emily sat there, mulling this over. "If I'm in charge of the money, I can make sure that the kids get what they need and want. My parents are always arguing with the number of things I buy for my kids. But they don't understand that I never wanted my son and daughter to go through what I did as a child." Marti nodded. "So it's important to you to have control of the money so you can make sure that no one goes without!" Emily's smile acknowledged that. Marti continued. "I can understand why it would be so scary for you to give up that control, especially if you quit work and go back to school."

Agreeing with Marti, Emily said, "I haven't depended on anyone like that since I left home. I don't know if I'll be able to do it, even if in the end it means that I'd have a more rewarding career."

Remembering Emily's earlier comments, Marti decided to push her a little more by asking, "Sounds like the thought of depending upon your husband brings up a lot of feelings." Emily took the bait, saying, "He'll be in charge. I'll probably have to justify everything I spend, even if it's for the kids. We'll have to watch every penny." Reflecting on what she'd just said, Emily added, "Just like my parents – except I won't be able to keep my mouth shut. There'll probably be a lot of arguing unless I just give up and go without."

There's that phrase again, thought Marti. So when Emily stopped, Marti tried to tie things together by asking, "Are you saying that depending upon your husband financially and not having total control of the budget is frightening to you because your life will be controlled by someone who might make you go without? Do you fear re-experiencing feelings of that unrelenting hunger because there isn't enough?"

"Yes," Emily lamented, "and I don't ever, ever want to go through that again."

Seeing the glistening in her eyes, Marti asked, "What's going on now?" Letting the tears roll down her cheeks, Emily said, "It was horrible. No matter what I did, I couldn't change things. I couldn't change them. My parents came from families that never showed affection, so we never got hugs or praise for our accomplishments. I thought if I was thin, then maybe they'd be different and love me. But I couldn't lose the weight." Reaching across the table for a tissue, she fell silent. On Marti's desk, the clock gave a soft chime as everyone waited. Marti spoke up, asking, "What did you feel?"

Taking a deep breath, Emily replied, "I just always felt that there was something wrong with me." The shame and humiliation that went with her memories could be seen in the sag of her shoulders. She didn't like feeling this way, but she had a new thought that brought some comfort: Marti would help her get through this. This newfound trust kept her from falling into the deep hole of despair that always accompanied these feelings. Except, she wished Marti would say something soon.

Right on cue, Marti said, "The truth is, I can't imagine that any child in your family would come away feeling loved or nurtured. Emily, you did not fail – you are not defective, or unlovable. Your parents for their own reasons could not give you what you needed, and you were so starved that the thought of going without what little food you had was too overwhelming. It was a matter of survival, and I'm proud of that little girl doing the only thing she could to survive." Then came a question. "Is it possible, Emily, that as a child, food took on another meaning; that it came to represent love – the love that was withheld from you – the love that you had to go without?" Tearfully, Emily nodded that this was true.

"And because of that," Marti said, "you always see to it that everyone else has enough – more than enough. The question is, do YOU know that there's enough food, time, and money – just for you?"

Again, Emily felt like she'd been jerked into a new dimension. Everything looked slightly different than before. "I guess not," she said. Marti explained, "I can see that going without time and money brings up the same feelings as when you go without food. So it will be vital for you to make sure that you always have enough. That means enough of the food that you like, enough money to buy the things you need and want, and enough time to eat when you are hungry, and rest when you are tired. Food is not going to make those hungers go away." Emily, feeling like she'd been on a roller coaster, sagged in her chair, saying, "All that is a lot to think about!"

Recognizing Emily's sudden droop as retreat, Marti knew that she'd assimilated all that she could for tonight. But, although Emily looked as if she'd had more than enough, she was beginning to understand herself better. Knowing causes and effects opened a door for her that she hadn't known existed just 20 minutes ago! Seeing that Emily was finished, Margaret wanted to speak but felt a little guilty taking center stage when Emily might have needed more time. But she knew that Marti wanted everyone to stick to their time limits, and everyone understood that. Everyone came to group knowing that they would have their turn to talk. So she said, "Bob and I have been through many phases with our finances. Now, he's in charge of our investments, savings account, and retirement funds. I'm in charge of all the household expenses. When he gets paid, he deposits some money into our joint checking account. The rest goes into savings. We meet regularly with a financial advisor who helps us plan our investments, and then Bob takes it from there. The only time in recent years when we had a problem was when I decided to redo that room. It occurred to me after Group a couple of weeks ago that we don't have fights or arguments about money because I never disagree with him. All these years, my life revolved around Bob, the boys, and their happiness. Now, it's my turn!" This was said with great confidence, an attitude everyone noticed. Continuing, Margaret said, "I sound tough here. But at home I have to fight the urge to be accommodating when I want something important. But, I'm happy to report that I've finished my room – and I love it! Sometimes I go in and close the door and just enjoy knowing that no one is going to interrupt me. Other times, I leave the door open and if Bob is home, he finds a reason to come in. He's even found reasons to stay awhile. That isn't something that I'd like all the time: it's my room, after all," she stated, obviously pleased with having established some boundaries. "But a visit once in awhile is nice."

Continuing, Margaret said, "You won't believe what happened a couple of days ago – Bob and I were in my room talking and out of the blue he asked me if I had thought about redecorating the rest of the house. I was so surprised, I didn't know what to say. Then he told me that compared to the rest of the house, he could understand why I retreated to my room. All these years I thought I knew what he liked – and he was thinking that I'd decorated the house with colors and furniture that I liked. Neither of us ever said a word. He wants me to go through each room and sketch my ideas for updating them. My mind has been spinning ever since. I've gone through the rooms, and the first thing I want to change are the colors;

they've always been too dark for me. There's so much to do: furniture, floors, painting. I'm even thinking about French doors in the family room." The speed of her words was increasing as she got caught up in the excitement of it all. "I might even redo my kitchen," she said, sounding thrilled with the opportunity. "I hope my husband knows how much this is going to cost! I can't wait to start shopping."

While everyone else chuckled, Julie was away in her thoughts, trying to imagine what it would be like to be in Margaret's position. Then Margaret's voice interrupted her wondering. She was answering Marti's question about food.

"One thing I can't figure out is why I felt so hungry after Bob and I talked about redecorating the house. I know it wasn't a physical hunger because we'd just finished dinner. And I've been grazing ever since." Marti jumped right in to ask, "What feelings came up when Bob mentioned changing the house?"

Even though she'd expected a question about feelings, Margaret did not have a ready answer. Oddly hesitant, she took a few moments to reply. "I started out being excited; pleased that he trusted my judgment and taste. But when he left the room a few minutes later, I found myself feeling kind of empty. Heaven only knows why!"

"Could it be that something Bob said upset you?" asked Marti.

Margaret took time to think back. What had Bob said? Finally, she said, "The only thing I can think of is when he told me to sketch my ideas, I felt different." Pleased to see Margaret making this connection, Marti inquired, "How different?" Uneasy, now, because she sensed that she was on the verge of discovering something important, Margaret squirmed. Did she want to know this or not? Recognizing it as internal pressure, not pressure from Marti or the Group, Margaret knew that it was time to get it out in the open. "Like someone had let the air out of my balloon," she said. Knowing that Margaret was so close, Marti asked, "Could it be that when the idea came up, you were thrilled because your creativity was unleashed –

like someone had just given you a blank canvas and a blank check. But when Bob wanted a sketch, it switched your attention from your ideas to wondering what he wanted in those sketches. Did he want every little detail, or did you have free reign? You couldn't help but wonder what would make him happy." Knowing that Margaret had almost gotten it, Marti instructed, "Listen to what you just said: your attention shifted from you to him." Then she waited. What would Margaret say to that?

Everyone watched Margaret catch herself. "I did it again, didn't I?" she asked them. Everyone nodded. Then Margaret could see it, too; she'd gone back to trying to second guess what Bob might want. In doing that, she'd left herself out of the picture. Satisfied, Marti said, "Very good; it's so easy to fall back on an old mind-set. It's going to be a challenge for you to change that because all these years your focus has been on pleasing everyone else. All that time you've made assumptions about what would make them happy. We don't know what Bob wants, but somehow you heard 'Do it the way I want,' not 'Do it the way you want'. So, the point is that it's not one or the other, but both of you sitting together and creating a environment to satisfy each of you. In the past when you were left out of the decisions, it made you feel deprived so you ate." Torn between elation that so much had been revealed and overwhelmed with the complexities involved, Margaret said, "This is all a lot more complicated than I thought!" The murmur around the table indicated that this was true for each of them as Marti said, "We have one more to go," and everyone turned to Kate.

Kate was feeling a little anxious. Having met with Marti individually a couple of times, Kate wondered if the therapist would mention their meetings. How would Marti use that information? Should SHE say something first? Deciding not to, she said, "I took a hard look at all this money stuff. I'm the one whose in charge of the money both at home and in the business. When we started out, Ed handled everything, but every time he bounced a check, he blamed it on me. We fought about money all the time. I don't remember how or when I took over, but I've been doing it for years."

"You mean he just dumped the whole thing on you?" Julie asked.

"Yup, but I like it better that way. I can't really trust him to pay the bills and keep our credit rating up. As long as he has enough spending money, good credit isn't important to him. But it is to me."

Kate sighed. To herself, she thought how difficult it had been to follow up on Marti's suggestion that she take an even closer look at her finances. It was even harder, she thought, to have to talk about it. "I have charge accounts at all the major stores," she said, feeling a little like she was in a confessional. "I have two VISAs, a Mastercard, and an American Express card. Basically the only debts we have are the house, the cars, and a line of credit. Ed, of course, has his own credit card, his tab at the bar, and his monthly bill at the liquor store. The biggest worry I have every month is 'the big unknown' – how much Ed run up on his personal accounts." Emily was appalled. Having a husband who was so secretive would drive her crazy.

"We have a savings account for the business," Kate was saying, "but our personal savings are zilch. I constantly worry about what would happen to our business if Ed disappeared again, or we split up."

It was running through everyone else's mind that she could run the business alone. Kate sounded like she had to have a husband to have a business and an income. Believing that to be true, Kate went on. "Ed and I spend a lot of money." Admitting this came slowly to Kate. On an even more personal level, she said, "I have a beautiful house, gorgeous furnishings, lots of clothes, a thriving business, but the truth of the matter is that we may be on the verge of losing it all." Stunned, everyone stiffened.

At the same time, Marti was thinking how good it was for Kate to risk opening herself up to possible criticism. So she smiled at Kate to show her support. Reinforced, Kate went on. "I really never looked at our money because I was afraid of what I would find. Then, too, I was afraid that I wouldn't know how to handle it. But I know now that if anything is going to change, I'm going to have to examine it. So, here's the rest of the story." The others, knowing how difficult this was for Kate, gave her encouraging smiles. Leaning forward as she continued, they listened intently. "Ed's not the only problem. I love to shop. It's like a hobby for me. If I'm not cruising the malls, I'm watching the shopping channel. What really gets me going are the sales. There's nothing like a good bargain."

Everyone wanted to ask questions, such as what are you buying? How much are you buying? Do you use any of it? When Kate paused, Emily was puzzled enough to ask. "Are you saying that shopping is a problem for you?"

"Maybe. Sometimes when I'm at the mall, I can almost forget that I have all these problems. So I guess I do use it as a way of dealing with things."

Verbalizing this suddenly opened up a new awareness for Kate. "I always go shopping after a fight. When the stores are closed, I watch the shopping channel." To herself, Kate thought that it was out now. They all probably think I should go to shoppers-anonymous. Marti's next question pulled her away from those thoughts. "Are you seeing a similarity here between what you do with shopping and what you do with food?"

"Well, I use both of them to make myself feel better. They distract me from whatever is going on. But it's not working any more. I haven't lost any more weight, and I can't keep up with the bills. It's gotten to the point where I have to take money out of our line of credit just to pay them. Ed doesn't know how bad off we are." Kate couldn't keep the bitterness out of her voice. "And I don't think he cares."

Now, everyone knew that Kate was in a financial crisis and was facing it all alone. Coming from common ground, Bobbie said, "You must be really worried!"

"It's the pits," Kate agreed.

Marti, suspecting that there was more involved, continued. "What happens when you know it's time to pay all those bills and there isn't enough money?" Kate took a minute to answer. "Before I even open the envelopes, I have this gigantic urge to buy something for myself," she said.

Marti asked, "Why's that?"

Kate took a minute to think that over. "I know we're going to be short again this month. And who knows how much he's spent on booze? It makes me want to buy what I want while I can because if I don't he's just going to drink it all up."

Marti said, "As you were talking I saw you with this beautifully decorated cake. You've just noticed that it has a piece missing, and you know that it is Ed who has eaten it. Knowing that he will soon be back for more, you feel it's urgent to eat as much as you can before he gets there. Otherwise, he'll eat it all up and there'll be nothing left for you."

She'd hardly finished when Kate was saying, "That's exactly it; damn him, he'll eat the whole thing!" Having felt the same way often enough, everyone chuckled. Encouraged, Kate added, "He lives like he's a swinging single – he never thinks how his actions affect me."

Marti was pleased with Kate's increasing ability to notice her own reactions to what Ed did. So she said, "I can understand how frightening it must be to think he is going to consume everything so that nothing is left for you. There is no sharing here. Seems like a lot of your spending is driven by fear rather than need."

Frowning, Kate said, "I never thought about that before, but I don't see how this is ever going to change: you know that I can't talk to him. These days he's never sober anyway. It's just hopeless."

Marti made a suggestion. "You might want to write this all up like a business plan so that Ed can understand that both of you are going to have to limit your spending or you will lose everything.

Somewhere, include a personal spending allotment." Kate's resistance could be heard in her answer. "I know that we'll end up in an argument because I'll be taking away his access to all of our money. What if he says he won't accept the plan?" Marti said, "My suggestion is to say something like 'Here are the financial facts. If you can figure a way around them, let me know. If you can't, we need to go to a financial advisor.'" Hearing this, Kate was less than confident that Marti's idea would work. But then, she'd never tried anything like this before, so maybe....

And then it was time for Marti to introduce the next assignment. Handing out the packets, she said, "This week we'll be looking at the feeling of anger and its relationship to food. For instance, after an argument with someone do you find yourself eating?" She went on to discuss anger, but no one was listening. Everyone was lost in their own thoughts.

CHAPTER EIGHT

I Have a Food for Every Feeling?

Week 17: Recognizing the Relationship Between Food & Anger

LOSING HER OFFICE WINDOW against the autumn chill, Marti glanced at her watch. Everyone should be in the reception room by now, and they were going to hear a repeat of what she'd said at the end of last week's session. It had been obvious, she remembered, that no one had heard a thing.

With a few minutes left, Marti reviewed notes she'd taken during a phone call received from Julie two days ago. Nearly hysterical, Julie had cried that she was sure Tom was going to divorce her. They'd had an enormous argument over finances, Julie said. Julie hadn't known how it occurred. According to her, she'd only explained her desire to know more about their finances, and she also wanted to have a percentage of her paycheck to spend as she wished. For some reason, Tom had gotten defensive, accusing her of not trusting him anymore. He'd also said that he didn't know why she was coming to Group when she hadn't lost any weight. But most of all, he hadn't understood why she wanted to change something that worked. Having said all that, he'd stormed from the house. What, Julie had asked, should she do?

Marti, now walking to the waiting room, remembered that she had tried to help Julie get beyond fears of divorce and abandonment, to see that this situation might have occurred because Tom was not yet used to the changes taking place within her. It had been Marti's suggestion that she continue talking with Tom to clarify any misunderstandings. The changes that Julie wanted had nothing to do, after all, with distrust. Catching a glance from Julie as she opened the door, Marti knew that something had happened. She could hardly wait to find out what it was.

When everyone was settled in their chairs, Marti was the first to speak. "The main focus over the last few weeks has been to create an environment for each of you that will support your weight loss and any other changes you may need or want to make in your lives. A big part of this involves feeling safe and secure. To do this, you will need to set boundaries and limits with others. 'No' is a word that is used to help define a personal boundary. Anger is a natural feeling that is experienced when that personal boundary is violated. So, you can see why it is important to be able to identify this feeling in yourself.

"Many people do not see a difference between anger, rage, and hostility. To them, it's all the same feeling. As women brought up in families where anger was not expressed or acknowledged, we are given many messages, such as ladies do not get angry, and it's not good to express a feeling that might cause waves. Sometimes there's a strong message that keeping it to yourself will protect the family from looking bad. We learn to push our feelings, especially anger, down, deep down inside. And how do we do that?" Looking around the table Marti continued with, "Alcohol, drugs and…" The women were quick to pick up on the pause and shouted in unison, "FOOD!"

Marti smiled proudly and said, "Right! So when we don't express and communicate anger and then eat, we gain weight. Let's look more closely at this feeling we call anger. Anger is focused on the present – today – right now. It is a response to a very specific action, word, or behavior. It is not directed at someone personally, such as when we say 'You are a bad person.' The message with anger is very simple: 'Ouch that hurt! Please don't do that again!' People then understand what is expected of them in a relationship with you. With anger, you communicate an action to resolve a problem. It is a constructive feeling because it helps to protect you and your relationships."

Having been married to someone like Ed, Kate was still dubious. So she asked, "Anger is good?" Marti nodded, but Kate was not convinced. She continued with, "The anger I've seen always left a path of destruction, which doesn't sound like anything you've just described." Marti responded with, "What you're talking about is rage, which is unresolved anger that has been stuffed down and become distorted over time. As more anger is piled onto what is already there, pressure begins to build to keep the rage deep down inside. Then something happens and the rage is unleashed and explodes outward in the form of retaliation, revenge, or retribution, with the main purpose of hurting others and/or destroying everything in sight. These feelings are rooted in the past and are directed more personally to the other person. An example of this might be statements such as 'You always do this, you idiot! Can't you ever learn? What's wrong with you?' Sometimes the raging person appears out of control and it can be terrifying to those on the receiving end. Often, they feel that their lives are being threatened. With rage, no one ever knows what they've done to incur this wrath. Nothing ever gets resolved. All anyone knows is that they have crossed over some unspoken line. It's like walking through a minefield – careful with each step because the next one could bring on an explosion."

"The purpose of this assignment was to help each of you to become aware of your angry feelings and to identify ways you cope with those feelings. So", Marti asked, "who would like to start?"

The silence was broken by a voice saying, "I will." All eyes turned to Bobbie, who immediately stated, "I'm not looking forward to this fund-raiser at my sister's this weekend – I HATE those things. If you listened to my mom, you'd think this was the event of the century. It drives me nuts because for weeks before it's all she can talk about. What I hate most is that Mother always insists upon selecting my entire outfit, like I was 10 years old. Well, this time it's going to be different. I exchanged the dress she sent over for something I really liked. Mother doesn't have the faintest idea I've done this. I hope someone takes a picture of her face when I walk through the door." Hmm, Marti thought, noticing that others were pulling back in their chairs as Bobbie spoke. They were responding to a change in Bobbie's usual, professional demeanor. Obviously angry – and hurt – Bobbie's voice was louder and shrill, over the indignities she felt she'd suffered at her mother's hands. It was Julie, playing her old role as "the fixer" who broke in to defuse the feelings by asking, "So, what kind of dress did you get?"

Bobbie, excited to share her victory, replied, "I'm glad you asked because I was going to tell you anyway. I found this full-length, royal blue dress that falls from the shoulders to the floor. I love it – but Mother will think it's too plain and simple because there isn't a single sequin on it. I also got shoes to match, and I'm wearing the simple pearl necklace my grandmother left me. And," here Bobbie gave a dramatic pause, "I've made an appointment to have my hair cut, too." This was a big change, everyone knew.

"I'm really tired of my hair. I've worn it this way only to keep it out of my face at work." Using her hands to show where it was being cut, she said, "I want it straight and smooth, and down to about here." Her hands stopped mid-neck. Amused with Bobbie's rebelliousness, Julie said, "With your new hair and everything, your mother is really going to be surprised."

"I can't wait," Bobbie replied. "I'll know right away if she disapproves, because she sends signals that can't be ignored. She won't yell at me or anything, but I won't be able to stand the look I'll get from her. Maybe I'll just make my entrance, chat a little, shake a few hands, and disappear."

Look? Marti wondered. Is this how Bobbie's mother communicates feelings? So Marti asked, "Is that how you know that your mother is angry?" The question caught Bobbie by surprise. Then she replied, "I guess so. My mother never raises her voice at me. What she does is give you that look, then she gets tense and silent and ignores me like I don't exist. When she's mad at others, she makes critical remarks under her breath. As for my father – I've never seen him really angry except when Mother spent too much money. Most of the time, he acts like he doesn't know what's going on but, once in a while, I'll notice that he's really tense about something."

"So," Marti said, "your parents held their angry feelings inside and didn't talk about them – which made it hard because you never knew what made them feel that way." Bobbie nodded in agreement as Marti continued. "No wonder you are so quick to pick up on other people's tension," she said. "It was the only way you could tell if your parents were angry or not. Along with the silent treatment, your mother also punished you by withdrawing her attention, making you feel that she didn't love you anymore. The threat of losing her love taught you to keep any negative feelings about her to yourself – especially anger. So you haven't had much practice in expressing yourself when you're angry at someone close to you."

Listening to Marti, Bobbie couldn't stop all the thoughts suddenly flooding into her consciousness. When she was able to ask a question, she said, "I've always had a hard time enduring someone's anger, but I thought that was normal. So, when you were talking about anger and the threat of losing love, it suddenly dawned on me all the things I do to avoid those feelings – especially with Garth. I've done it so much that most of the time I don't even know it. People have asked me, 'Didn't that make you mad?' I always felt stupid saying that it hadn't – logically, it should have."

Bobbie was not alone – Margaret, Julie, and Emily were all in agreement and said that they, too, did not feel safe in feeling or expressing their anger. Kate, on the other hand, was still trying to figure out if she felt anger, or rage. So she sat silently, contemplating this.

Another thought occurred to Bobbie. "God – no wonder it took a whole week to realize that I was mad at Garth!" Going on, she told how he'd gone on a sales trip he'd won to Paris. Paris – the place they'd talked about visiting together. "I keep asking myself why he didn't invite me to go along – then I told myself that it was only for a week, and we wouldn't have time to see the things we said we wanted to see, anyway!"

Disbelief hung in the air. He hadn't invited her? Emily asked, "You mean, he could have taken you?"

"Yes," said Bobbie. "I would have had to pay my own airfare, but the hotel would have been free. And, I've got all sorts of vacation time coming." Seeing everyone else's shock loosened a knot deep inside of Bobbie that she hadn't known was there. Eyes glistening, she said, "I can't believe he would do this to me – he knew how much I wanted to go. We've talked about it. But now that I think about it, he never includes me in on any of his functions."

"Never?" asked Margaret. "Do you invite him to yours?"

"Yes," Bobbie replied, her voice suddenly brittle. "He'll be back in time to go to my sister's fund-raiser."

Marti, hearing a change in tone, said "Sounds like you're feeling angry. Do you have any other feelings?" Bobbie replied, "Well, I'm disappointed, of course." After a pause, she said, "And I guess I feel left out, too." Follc ing up on that, Marti asked, "And hurt?" Here, Bobbie eyes started to well up, again. "Yes," she said, tears rolling down her cheeks. "And I really don't know how to handle it – I'm so afraid that if I ask too much of Garth, he'll leave me."

Knowing that Bobbie would need some encouragement, Marti counseled, "It's okay to let yourself feel the hurt." After a few seconds, Bobbie wiped away her tears and Marti continued by asking, "What do you need or want that would help with this feeling?"

Bobbie allowed the others to see the full pain behind her eyes. Then she said, "I guess I need to know where my relationship with Garth is going. I need to know what his feelings are toward me. Are we a couple, or not?"

Marti could see that Bobbie and the others were beginning to learn that feelings were not to be avoided because they are the key to resolving problems. Feelings open the door to needs and wants which then lead to resolution. In this process, food begins to lose its soothing power. But the Group was still focused on Bobbie's immediate dilemma. "So what are you going to do?" Margaret asked.

"I guess I need to talk to him," Bobbie said in a whisper. "But I'm not sure I know what to say to him – especially since we haven't yet resolved our money issues." Marti then suggested role-playing. "Bobbie, there are two ways to communicate. One is to be aggressive, which never resolves anything. The other is to be assertive, which allows you to express what you are feeling in a way that the other person can hear it. So let's practice. You be Garth and I will be you."

As Bobbie went through this demonstration, she began to hear the different responses she could give to anything Garth might say. The selection of words and the practice she received in communicating them began to make her more confident about how she was going to present this sensitive topic.

When they were through practicing, Bobbie summarized aloud, "I think I can do it – I'll ask where he sees our relationship going, and I'm going to tell him what I think is working and not working. Maybe he'll agree, and then our relationship will be different. I guess I'll find a way to deal with it if he decides to leave, because I can't go on living with someone who isn't committed to being in a relationship with me." Bobbie was relieved that she could actually see herself doing this without getting into a huge argument and… maybe she could survive losing Garth.

Listening, Marti said, "Good for you." To herself, she noted how much progress Bobbie was making in standing up to the people in her life. Then Julie, noticing that it was time for the next person, said, "I'll go next."

"It's been another upsetting week. I tried really hard to present my ideas to Tom about my being more involved in our finances and we ended up in a huge fight. For the first time in our marriage, he walked out on me – I was sure he was never coming back. After about an hour, I called Marti. She assured me that he'd be back eventually, and when he did, she said I should I try to clarify any misunderstandings. Well, she was right – he did come back. And before I lost my courage, I told him that I didn't mean to upset him, or make him feel that he was doing something wrong, I just wanted to be more informed about our finances – and I didn't want to have to ask for his permission to buy every little thing." Her demeanor showing how surprised she'd been at his reaction, she said, "It turned out great. His attitude changed and we talked. Then he took me downstairs and showed me which program on the computer had all our financial information. He was kind of impressed with how fast I learned to use it." Proudly, she said, "I'm really amazed at how well he's done with our money. Here I thought we didn't have very much, but he's done very well with our investments and savings. Now I understand why he spends so much time on the computer."

When everyone expressed their pleasure at Julie's working things out, she countered it by saying, "There's more. The other thing that happened is that my mother left another message telling me that my brother's back. Nobody's knows where he's been, or what he's been doing. Mom finished with, 'Thanks for all your help,' which I know she didn't mean. Then she hung up. I decided not to respond to that, either. I wasn't looking forward to my birthday last Friday. I guess she tried to get back at me by not sending a card or anything. Tom and the kids and I celebrated my birthday alone, and you know, it was wonderful! For the first time, there wasn't anyone there to ruin it. That's when I realized how peaceful my life has become since I stopped responding to my mom and brother and their expectations. I really don't want to do that anymore. They're never going to change, anyway. But it makes me feel bad when I tell you this because daughters aren't supposed to talk about their mothers like that."

Marti objected, "Your mother says and does things that hurt you, and you have every right to be upset by them. It sounds like you are beginning to recognize the games your mother plays to avoid her own anger and other feelings, too. Making you the scapegoat somehow makes her feel better." Julie nodded. "Anger is a really hard feeling for me to look at," she said. "My brother and I grew up with my grandmother after my parents divorced. She was always angry or maybe it was rage. To hear her tell it, we never did anything right. Because my mother was either at work or dating, she was never there. Grandmother took it out on us by restricting us to our rooms. Our only escape was to go outside – and that's when my brother got into drugs, leaving me all alone to deal with her tirades. Sometimes it was something that my mom did, other times we'd done something. But, whatever it was, I knew that I was going straight to hell. Even when she was at home, Mom never stood up to my grandmother, not even to protect us. Seeing us as heathens, Grandmother was scared to death I'd grow up like my mother – who'd been divorced by my father when he found her in bed with another man. I was eight years old when my parents divorced, but I can still remember my parents fighting. Mom had a way of baiting him and he would respond by yelling back at her. Then mom would break dishes, or slam doors, and he'd punch his hand through the wall, or drive off squealing his wheels."

Marti commented to the Group, "What Julie witnessed between her parents was rage, not anger. And it's a good example of how destructive rage can be. What you saw as a child is that rage not anger breaks families apart. Somehow from all of this, you got a message that it was your responsibility to take care of everyone – especially your mother and her feelings."

To herself, Marti was thinking that Julie probably has many angry feelings toward both her parents; her mother for not protecting her, and leaving her with her grandmother, and her father for not taking responsibility for his children.

"My mom has always been an angry person," Julie went on to say. "except when she was 'in love.' Then she was just gone. Between affairs, she was too busy for us."

"How does all this affect your ability to express anger now?" Marti wanted to know.

"Well, for one thing, I married someone who was not an angry person. My husband and I rarely have arguments, and we've never had fights like my parents."

Emily asked, "So do you always agree on everything?"

"No. It just means that I'm careful to remind myself that whatever we're discussing is not worth fighting over."

"What happens to the feelings that you don't express?" queried Marti.

"I keep them to myself," Julie answered.

"And then what happens?" Marti asked.

Before Julie could think it over, the words popped out of her mouth. "I eat," she said. Listening to her own words, she realized just how often she ate in response to her feelings. Kate said, "Well, you're not alone!" And everyone else nodded.

Marti pressed on. "So, what you're saying is that you get upset about something, you don't want to say anything because it might lead to a big fight – and maybe then – the fight would eventually lead to a divorce. So, you keep your feelings to yourself, and you eat, and then you gain weight."

"Well, when you say it that way," Julie said, "it seems like a lot of things I do or don't do result in eating. No wonder my body's in this shape. It just seems that there's so much to do that I don't know if I can do it."

"I can understand why you may be feeling a little overwhelmed right now," Marti said. "The adults in your life didn't take the time – or didn't know how – to talk about feelings. So, you don't know, because you were never taught. Now that you are more conscious about your food, and not using it to bury your feelings, you are more aware of the times when you do feel anger, disappointment, etc. And you are also learning new ways to more accurately take care of those feelings. But this is unknown territory, and that in itself can be overwhelming. I promise you, Julie, that as you keep working, this overwhelming feeling will go away."

It was the end of her turn, but Julie was thinking anew of her grandmother, her mother, and brother. No one, Julie knew, would ever understand how she felt about the people in her family. Now that she had this new awareness of herself and how others affected her, it was hard to accept that her true feelings about them amounted to wishing that they weren't in her life. But they were, so she decided that she had to deal with it.

It was Kate's turn. "While you guys were talking, I was thinking that I'd lived with anger every day of my life. Then you told the difference between rage and anger and I suddenly realized that I've been dealing with rage all along. But I didn't know that last week when I was trying to get the courage to approach Ed with our money crisis. Before talking to him, I'd decided that he would accept the news better from a financial advisor. So I made an appointment and brought all the information in for a professional evaluation. Then I thought it would be safer to bring up the subject in a public place, so I took the report to his favorite bar and grill when I knew that he'd be there. It was early enough that he'd only had his morning eye-opener, which means he was in a relatively good mood. When I went in, I handed him the report. He read it because, otherwise, he'd have to talk to me.

"Of course, he didn't want to believe it. He sat there, reading it and holding his head in his hands. He was swearing under his breath. I was on pins and needles, waiting for him to blow up. Then he looked up at me and I could see that he was furious. 'What the hell happened, here?' he hissed at me. 'Why didn't you tell me, earlier, you fat bitch. I knew I shouldn't have trusted you!' I interrupted him by handing him a list of five ways that would help turn things around. When he saw that we were both going to have to give up our credit cards, I was giving up the shopping channel, he was going to have to stop running up tabs and credit at the liquor store, but we would each receive a set amount of cash each month, he actually agreed. I was so relieved. Who would have expected him to agree? Yet, I knew that this probably wouldn't last long. And I was right. Two nights later, I got a call from the police station. Ed had torn up a bar after finding out that his tab had been canceled. Then he tried to drive off. The bartender called the police and they arrested him half a mile away. He would have been farther, but he was too far gone to know where he was going. This was his third or fourth DUI, so they took him to jail and he called me. I told him that I would call our lawyer, but I wasn't going to bail him out this time. When he started in on me, I just hung up – I knew that it would make him madder, but I didn't care. The police would have to deal with it, not me. At least for now. When I finally got hold of the attorney, he said he would take care of everything. He's going to recommend that Ed go into a drug and alcohol rehab program. But I don't know if Ed will do it because he doesn't think he has a problem, and he's refused to go before. But, then again, this time he may not have a choice."

Margaret couldn't help but break in. "Kate, I had no idea things were that bad." Emily followed up with, "I can't believe that you've been living this way for so long." Then Marti asked, "What about you, Kate? What happened to you while all this was going on?" It didn't take Kate long to say, "I started remembering my alcoholic father. Nothing worked for him – not jail, or AA. Every time he got into trouble, he promised that he'd quit drinking. But he didn't. He'd go back to drinking after work, then come home and start yelling at us. Pretty soon, he was violent again. We all knew that someone was going to get hurt, and it was usually Mom. So, when he started after her, she'd yell for me to call the police. And when dad got home from jail, he'd beat me up for calling the cops – as if it was all my fault. In our house, we walked on eggshells whenever Dad was around. We had to be careful not to set him off. The awful thing is that we never knew what would do that!"

Knowing what it was like to come from abusive families, Emily and Julie could really understand Kate's sadness. As a Group, everyone was beginning to understand that their weight hadn't just happened because of failed diets and lack of willpower. No wonder, thought Bobbie, that it's taking so long to lose the weight: its roots started back when we were all little girls.

Continuing, Kate was admitting, "Ed drinks a lot, too, but until the other night, I didn't think he'd be violent. When the boys were young, he slapped them and me around a couple of times, but nothing like my dad who beat us. Now I realize that Ed and my dad aren't so different after all. I hope he goes to rehab, because I don't know that I can live with a man like my father. It makes me angry just realizing how much alike they are. But there's nothing I can do about it and that's when I eat."

"Anything in particular?" Marti inquired.

"Now that you ask, I like to eat things I can bite and crunch, like chips," Kate replied, wondering why Marti wanted to know.

Marti said to the group, "This is a really good example of figuring out what kinds of foods go with what feelings. For Kate, when she's really angry, but feels helpless to fix it, she'll have an urge for crunchy foods." Then talking directly to Kate she continued, "So, next time you have a craving for chips or crunchy food, you will be reminded to check with your body. If you are not eating for physical hunger, then you may be eating for anger. Returning her attention

to the group Marti stated, "Specific foods can be a cue for unconscious eating. All of you will be able to identify these foods as you
become more aware of your feelings."

Kate asked, "How do you talk to someone who yells and screams
all the time?" Marti replied, "It is very challenging to talk to someone who is doing everything he can not to hear what you have to
say. The only thing I can suggest is to stay focused on your message,
making sure you are doing everything you can to present it in a
non-threatening way. Earlier, I mentioned aggressive and assertive
communication. This might be a good time to explain in more
detail, the difference between the two. Kate, it would not surprise
me if you have adopted a more aggressive style because of your constant exposure to rage and hostility. You've always had to be alert so
that you could defend yourself. And that's one of the key differences. Aggression is experienced as an attack. It never resolves anything because both parties feel they have to defend themselves. You
are reacting to one another rather than communicating the real
issues.

On the other hand, communicating assertively means that each
person takes responsibility for his or her own feelings. It's not about
what 'you' did wrong; it's about 'me', what I feel, and what I want or
need to change. So the other person understands, in the end, how
their actions affected you and what they can do in the future to prevent doing it again. Kate, if Ed was sitting right here, what would
you want to say to him?" Not wasting a single second, Kate said,
"'You son of a bitch, look at what you've done. You're nothing but a
drunken, lazy, no-good bastard!'" Everyone burst into laugher and
cheers. Her words were so brutal – so honest. Marti asked, "Is Kate
expressing this assertively or aggressively?"

"Aggressively," everyone replied, still laughing.

At first, Kate laughed along with everyone else. Then her frustration returned, and her face grew more intense as she made another
attempt to express what she was feeling. "'You hurt me and I'm not

going to take it anymore. And if you don't like it, take a hike!'"

"Okay," Marti repeated, "would you call that presentation aggressive or assertive?"

Kate said, "Definitely aggressive. I just don't know how to say it any other way."

Pleased to see that Kate was getting it, Marti wanted to encourage her to take the next step. "The secret is that aggressive statements usually start with 'YOU,'" she said. "'You did this... you did that!' Assertive statements are 'I' statements. For example, another way of stating your point would be, 'I'm very unhappy with our relationship. It's not working for me. I've been hurt over and over again. I'm not ready to give up on us, but I've begun to make changes in myself, and I'm asking you to make some changes, too. I've decided not to be in a relationship where I don't feel loved and treasured and valued. If our relationship doesn't change, I will need to make other decisions.'"

Hearing this, Kate was deep in thought. This was so much less explosive, but it is very clear as to what's wrong, what needs to change, and what will happen if no change is made. It really did communicate better what she wanted to say. But she had to MEAN it before she said it, so it was scary. In other words, if he didn't make changes, she was going to have to leave him. "Well," she said, "I don't know when I'll get the chance to say anything to him. Maybe I'll get a chance to talk to him with the lawyer present. That way, maybe he'll be more open to what I have to say. And maybe that'll encourage him to try rehab. I just hope that I can do it."

Marti didn't want Kate ending on the phrase, "I just hope I can." It signified that Kate's old helplessness had taken over. Marti knew that this feeling would block any action, and nothing would change. So Marti needed to find a way to re-frame the task so Kate would be more able to take control of the situation. Making eye contact with Kate, Marti said, "The issue is not whether you can or cannot do it, because you CAN do it. The issue is believing that you are important enough to make the choice to take care of yourself!"

"What have you got to lose?" Bobbie asked, wanting to lend support.

Kate moved in her chair, as if having a hard time with all this encouragement. "You're right. At this point, I guess I have nothing to lose." Then it was Emily's turn.

Emily was still not her usual smiling self. That Emily had been steadily disappearing since her parents moved in. However, everyone was shocked to hear the defeat in her voice as she said, "Well, I had a terrible week. It's harder than ever to get my work done at the clinic. I called the university about getting my application in and found out that it has to be in by Monday. I don't know how I'm going to get everything together by then. On top of that, remember that I was going to ask my brother and sisters to take mom and dad for a meal now and then? Well, no one would take them right away. And I don't hold out much hope that they'll do it at all. But, they did tell me how much they appreciate what I'm doing for OUR parents. I know that they just aren't about to put themselves in a position where they could get stuck with them. So I'm left with my mother taking over my life. I'm feeling really threatened by this because it's interfering with everything I've learned in this program."

Everyone could see that this was a very big issue. With every minute, tension was building in Emily's body as she continued. "I'm really worried because I'm noticing a drastic change in ME, and how I eat now that my parents are around. I know that I've gained weight and that makes me feel even worse because I know that I'd lost weight before they moved in. I feel like a child again, like I have no control over my life."

Emily was relieved that no one could hear what was going on inside of her. A little-girl's voice was screaming as loud as it could, "I hate them, I hate them," over and over again. The sound of Marti's voice caught Emily's attention. "What feelings come up as you're talking about this?" Her voice haggard, Emily said, "I'm feeling trapped. I can't stand what my mother is doing to me, and my father just sits there like he agrees with her. My kids are constantly hungry. I'm hiding food again and eating in the bathroom. My husband knows that I'm upset, but he doesn't know why. Besides, he wouldn't know what to do. He tries to make me feel better by reminding me that they'll be gone soon. He thinks he's helping, but that's not what I need at all."

"So what do you need?" Marti inquired.

"I need for my parents to stop treating me like a child," Emily replied.

"What are you going to do?" Julie asked, concern written all over her face.

With a look of dread, Emily said. "I'm going to have to talk to them about it," she said. "It won't be easy because I've never done anything like this before." It was not unusual, Marti knew, for adults to return to childhood communication patterns with their parents. So Marti jumped at the opportunity to role-play. Before she could say anything, Bobbie was already suggesting it. Having experienced the benefits of it herself, Bobbie asked, "Would it help to practice?" Emily nodded, and that was all Bobbie needed. "Pretend," she said, "that I'm your mom and I've just served you." Bobbie was on her feet, acting like she'd just put a plate down in front of Emily. "Emily," she said, "Here's your special food. I fixed it just for you because I know that you want to lose weight."

Forcefully, Emily replied, "It's none of your business what I eat. My weight is my business, not yours." Pausing to gulp away nervousness, Emily continued, "I'm not a child anymore. This is my kitchen, and you are a guest in MY house. So stop cooking and cleaning. Stop treating me like I don't know what I'm doing, and stop telling me what's best for me."

"Wow," said Marti. "You sound really angry at your Mom." Everyone nodded their heads. Glad to have Marti take over, Bobbie sat down.

Marti had been writing down Emily's words so they could edit them, if needed. She read them back to Emily, asking, "Would this be aggressive or assertive communication?"

"Well, when you read it to me, it sounded like an attack," commented Emily.

"You're right. Your mother will be so busy defending herself that she won't be able to hear what you have to say. So let's go back and look at another way of saying the same things." To give her an example, Marti said, "How would it be if you said, 'Mother, I'm unhappy with the way things are going between us. I need to tell you that your comments about my weight and my food are not helping me. In fact, they hurt me very deeply – and it needs to stop. My weight is no longer open for discussion.'"

Emily couldn't picture herself saying anything like this to her mother. Sure, she'd sounded tough a minute ago, but that's because she was safe here. So she said, "It sounds good, but I can't do it. It's too scary."

Marti, feeling the resistance, decided to take a different approach. So she continued with, "I'm not asking this of your little girl – because you are no longer a little girl. When you were a child, you couldn't talk back to your parents. But now you're all grown up and you have your own house and kids, so the adult part of you needs to be present when you are around your mother and to teach your mother what is expected of her if she is to have a healthy adult/adult relationship with you. So visualize yourself talking to your mother from your strong, adult place. Then the adult can deal with her." But Emily found that her little girl had come back in the middle of this. What if her mother exploded? If she upset her mother, her father would be mad, too. What if they just stormed out and never came back. How could she survive without them? Emily sighed and said to herself that she guessed she'd just cross that bridge when she got to it. Then it was Margaret's turn.

Margaret started off by saying, "Well, I'm having a great time with my project. The painters have been there all week. I can't believe the difference a coat of paint can make. My husband noticed right away. I've tried to involve him more by talking about it, but he's not that interested. So I'm doing it the way I want – which is probably the way he wanted in the first place. My son hasn't noticed anything, but it probably has to do with what happened last week. With all the confusion and work around the house, it was Donnie's turn to have Devon stay with us. Only, he had other plans. By the time he got around to her, they had maybe an hour together. Here his little girl comes to visit him and he just assumes that because I'm there, I'll take care of her. It's not that I don't want to, she's an angel, I just hate to see her so disappointed when he's off doing something else. I'm really disappointed in him. I think my son should be more responsible, especially where his daughter is concerned. So I talked to him, and he seemed to know what I was saying and said that he'd take care of it. But his idea of taking care of it when Devon came this last weekend was to ask me to take care of her while he went out with his buddies."

"But I thought you said what upset you is that he doesn't spend time with his daughter," Kate remarked.

Margaret's reaction surprised everyone. "Don't you think that upset is too strong a word?" she asked. "I wasn't upset, maybe a little annoyed."

"Annoyed?" Julie asked. Emily said, "Margaret, you told us that he frequently leaves his daughter to go off and play. Then his daughter is disappointed that she doesn't have more time with him."

"Okay," Margaret said, "maybe I'm a little irritated."

Knowing that Margaret needed help in identifying her anger, Marti said, "Margaret, it seems hard for you to identify the exact feeling when your son continues to ignore his responsibilities with his daughter, which ends up hurting her and brings up feelings in you, too. If you're really feeling angry, but you treat it as an irritation, nothing ever gets resolved. That could lead to feeling deprived.

And what happens when you feel deprived?" Together, everyone said, "You eat!"

An alarm went off in Margaret's head. Could there be another reason for her weight gain. What if it wasn't all memories, abuse, and trauma. What if it had to do with... she couldn't keep quiet any longer. "I used to think that my sudden gain over the past two years was over the abuse. Now I'm wondering if my son's move back home two years ago could be a part of it too."

Marti was impressed with Margaret's newfound insight. She responded with, "It's very possible. What are you feeling right now?"

"Well," Margaret said, "let me assure you that it's not irritation." Here, she paused. Pursing her lips in concentration, she took time to get in touch with the depth of her feelings. Almost as if she was embarrassed that she could feel that negative about anything, she said, "I guess it's anger because, all of a sudden I want to kick Donnie out. I'm absolutely furious!" Then, aghast at what she'd just said, Margaret clapped her hand over her mouth as if to push the words back. "I can't believe I said that; I didn't know that I was that angry at Donnie," she said. "Can you tell us a little more about that feeling, Margaret?" Marti asked.

"He's my son and I love him, but when does my job as a mother ever end?" Turning to the rest of them Margaret said, "I haven't worked outside my house like the rest of you because I wanted to stay home to be a full-time mom. I really enjoyed it, and I have no regrets. But now, it's my turn. I don't know what that means yet, but I do know that it's not taking care of my adult sons, or their children, on a full time basis!"

"Way to go!" Kate cheered. Julie actually clapped very quietly.

Suddenly Margaret felt guilty. What kind of a mother was she, anyway? "I don't know if I really want to kick him out. Where would he go? He'd hate me and maybe he'd never come back. Then I wouldn't see Devon, either. No, I just couldn't do that."

"Well, what else could you choose to do?" asked Marti.

"I could talk to him, but I already tried that and it went nowhere."

"Does your son work?" Bobbie asked, wondering what else was going on here.

"Part-time," Margaret replied. "After his marriage failed, he decided to get his MBA and went back to school. When he came to us for help, we decided to let him move back home. I felt so bad for him." Then, deciding to tell all, she continued, "With the money he makes from his job, he pays for school and some of his bills. There's nothing left for child support, so my husband and I have been helping with that, too."

"So he doesn't pay rent?" Emily asked.

Kate was thinking about her own boys when she added, "And he doesn't have any chores to do because he's never home!" To herself, Marti was saying, that this introduced an area that Margaret may have other feelings about money. She could see in Margaret's words and body language that she had some strong feelings about it. Getting to them, Marti said, "What's going on inside, Margaret?"

"I guess," Margaret said, pausing a few seconds, "I guess I am feeling angry about everything!"

Knowing that they were getting somewhere, Marti acknowledged, "You have a lot of reasons for feeling angry, Margaret." To the rest of the Group, she said, "This is a good example of what happens when we fall back into old patterns without thinking about what we really want or need. The result of that unconscious decision-making process is what Margaret is feeling now – angry, trapped, used."

The others nodded in agreement.

"Now that you're aware of some of the things making you feel angry," Marti said, "what would you like to say to your son?"

"Well, he's working very hard and I don't want to make it more difficult. So I don't know what to say," Margaret replied, halfway hoping she wouldn't have to do anything.

Marti could hear that Margaret had hit the wall of resistance again. Knowing that this was part of the process, Marti wanted to help her work through it. So she said, "Telling him will do two things – first, he will know what you expect of him, and what the consequences will be if he oversteps your limits again. Second, you will be helping him to grow up by teaching him that an adult relationship is a two-way street: there's give and take from both sides."

Focusing on the words "adult relationship," it occurred to Margaret that Donnie's wife probably divorced him because she got tired of having a little boy for a husband. Having identified Donnie's problem, Margaret felt better. "I want to tell him that he has to be more responsible with Devon, and that he needs to move out when he graduates," she said. "I don't want to continue taking full responsibility for his support payments. His other bills have to have come down over two years, so he can start assuming part of the payment. I want to tell him that things are going to be different around the house. From now on, he can do his own laundry and take care of his own dry cleaning. And I'm going to stop giving him money for gas."

Everyone was shocked: she gave him gas money, too? "You have been really good to him for the past two years," said Emily. "But doing these things is the next step in getting him ready to be a full-time adult." Kate was saying to herself, "I wish my mother-in-law would have done something like that – maybe Ed would be more willing to be an adult."

Affirming everything Margaret had said, Marti commented, "You've explained your boundaries and limits beautifully to us. When you give them to your son, the only thing that I would change is that I'd put in a few I's." Margaret got out her pen and started writing. "For example, 'Don, I'm not happy with how things are working here, between you and me. I've given this a lot of thought, and I decided that we need to make some changes – some are immediate, others will occur over time. Starting today, I expect you to do your own laundry and dry cleaning, pay for your own gas, pick up after yourself in the kitchen, and – if you choose not to keep your room tidy – keep the door to your bedroom closed. Starting next month, Dad and I will be giving you half of what you pay now for child support because we think it's important that you begin to assume more financial responsibility for your child, especially since you will be graduating soon. That leads to the next thing that bothers me. I'm very disappointed in how you're handling your visitations with Devon. Your daughter is hurt when you don't spend time with her. She can't help but feel that you don't love her. I don't believe that you purposely want to hurt your child, so I hope you'll make some changes there too. And the last thing is that you will be graduating in June and I expect that you will have a job by that time, which will allow you to afford your own place and assume full responsibility for your child's support. This may sound harsh right now, but I hope you will take time to think about it. Then maybe you'll see that our intent has been, and always will be, to help you.' And, Margaret, you might want to talk this over with your husband because he has opinions of his own. Who knows, he might be supportive!"

Margaret was rushing to get every last word down in her journal. Feeling motivated by how much this would be helping everyone: Donnie, Devon, and herself, she was eager to do it. Then she could hear Marti continuing, "After you have finished your presentation, it will be good to give Donnie a chance to respond. So you could say something like, 'I've finished with what I needed to say, now it's your turn.' Then, based upon his response, you will work together to come to an agreement that works for both of you. This is called compromise, and the important thing about this is that each person feels satisfaction over the final agreement and your anger will be resolved."

Margaret knew that this was not going to be easy, mostly because she'd never done it before. Aloud, she said, "I hope I can do this because it's so important. I just hope that he doesn't take it wrong and go running off in anger." Marti had a quick response. "He'll come back, and then you can continue your talk. If he takes it wrong, stay with it until everything is clarified. The point is that by resolving anger, you build closer relationships. It doesn't have to stay stuffed down inside or, most importantly, you don't have to eat to make it go away. I'll bet you all never thought," and, here, Marti spoke to all of them, "that communicating your feelings would lead to weight loss."

There was fifteen minutes left in the session when Marti went to the tape machine and pushed a button. Suddenly, soft music filled the air and, like clockwork, everyone got up and moved their chairs back from the table, then reseated themselves in comfortable positions. Along with the soothing notes, Marti began to recite the words for their relaxation and visualization. They'd been doing this meditative exercise for the last five weeks, and it had become one of the highlights of the meetings. "I love this part." Emily said.

"I need it!" Kate exclaimed as everyone closed their eyes and felt their bodies begin to release all the tension and strain of the week. When they were brought back to the present, everyone felt rejuvenated. Before gathering up their belongings, Marti said, "I want to remind you that the last session of this group will be next week. I'd like everyone to think about whether or not they would like to continue to the next part of the program."

Kate asked, "What is the next part?"

"In Phase One, you were given tools to lose weight and maintain the loss, and you began to create an environment or lifestyle that supports your weight loss and other changes in your life. However, many women find that there are other blocks to losing weight. One of those blocks will be covered in the next phase. In Phase Two, we look at your negative, critical, judgmental thoughts and see how they are obstacles to making changes in your weight and life in general. You will learn how to change that inner chatter into a belief system that is more positive, supportive, and validating. We will also be working on body image, and how that affects weight loss. When someone has a bad body image, it feeds into all the negative judgments and beliefs about themselves. In other words, when you say 'I hate my body,' you are also saying you hate yourself! That makes losing weight more difficult – if not impossible."

Silence greeted her words, which wasn't surprising, she thought, given the fact that this might be a tough decision to make. So she began handing out next week's assignment, which called for them to assess at how they'd changed in the past eighteen weeks: how they ate, how they viewed food, how they were dealing with their feelings, and how they'd already changed their environment. Then she said, "Be thinking about changes in others as well as yourselves. And, bring in a sheet of your favorite notepaper next week." In answer to a few surprised glances, she said, "It will be a nice surprise!"

CHAPTER NINE

But Wait A Minute, I'm Not Done Yet!

Week 18: The End and The Decision

A WEEK LATER, in the light of a fading day, the five women returned for the final meeting in Phase One. Opening the door, Marti couldn't help but wish she had taken pictures of everyone 18 weeks ago. Then they would all see the transformation she saw. No one looked the same. Pleased, she smiled at each of them as her eyes swept around the room. That's when she noticed that Kate was a little withdrawn. Perhaps, Marti thought, Kate only appeared that way because the others were no longer so emotionally isolated. Nowadays, it was as if they were extending their individual spaces in an effort to include one another. Even with that, though, Marti sensed an uneasiness in them today. The last meeting was always filled with mixed emotions. As with all endings, it signaled a change. On one side of change there was a sense of achievement and predictability, and on the other fear and the unknown. Each woman was sitting with some anxiety, thinking about who was going to stay and who would leave. Goodbyes were always hard. But Marti knew that they were not ending anything. The breakthroughs initiated in Phase One had only introduced these women to what they could accomplish. Gaining additional access to what was going on inside of them during the next 20 weeks would allow them to get even closer to their own personal truths.

Once inside the conference room, Marti began. "I want to congratulate each of you for the tremendous changes you've made. The biggest change I've witnessed is the consciousness that each of you brings to what you're doing with food. You've discovered that you have a far wider range of choice in what you enjoy eating."

That's true, the five nodded, as Bobbie thought that she wasn't eating nearly the number of candy bars she used to. A few seats away, Julie was marveling that she no longer felt guilty about throwing table scraps away. Who would have believed that? she mused.

"Another change," Marti mentioned, "is that all of you now realize that losing weight is far more complicated than just what food you eat." Jokingly, she added, "CHOCOLATE is not the enemy!" Of all of them, Bobbie was most amused. Talk about a belief that's hard to get rid of! Continuing, Marti listed another of her observations. "It's obvious that you are all making conscious efforts to eat for physical hunger, which tells me that you are listening to your bodies more and can more easily identify the other hungers. I've seen all of you begin to find more accurate ways to take care of those other hungers. To support all of this, you've started creating environments that will sustain the changes in your bodies and lives. So with these tools and lifestyle changes, you've laid the foundation you need to lose weight and maintain weight loss. However, most women feel that with all this accomplished, their work has only just begun. I want to tell you what comes next."

To this point, all five had been fully engrossed in what Marti was saying. Now, however, Kate found herself pulling back. It was true that she'd made a number of changes, and maybe she could have made more if she'd attended regularly. But, still....

"You will continue doing what you started in Phase One," Marti explained. "In addition, in Phase Two, we will be focusing on the negative, critical, and judgmental thoughts that have in the past blocked you from losing weight and/or keeping it off. We will be showing you ways to change those thoughts to more positive, nurturing, and supportive ones. With this change you will find your beliefs and attitudes changing and will no longer feel 'stuck.' Then your energies will be freed to move your life in more fulfilling directions. We will also be working on your perceived and real body images, picturing your body as it is now and at your natural body weight." Seeing Emily frowning, Marti explained further.

"Visualizing your body at different weights will help to bring up other fears and blocks to losing weight. In Phase One, we worked on creating a safe external environment to support and nurture change. In Phase Two, you will begin to create a safe internal environment to sustain change. So," she said, smiling. "I'd like to go around and find out what's happened this past week, and then you can tell me what you've decided about going on to Phase Two. Who would like to go first?" Before Marti was through asking the question, Bobbie's hand was in the air. Marti couldn't help but notice Bobbie's new hairdo. There was something else, too – a certain sparkle in her eyes.

Bobbie was bursting to tell them all that had happened. Leaning eagerly forward in her seat, she started with, "Notice anything different?" Then, playfully, she turned her head side to side to set her hair swinging. "I hope you like it because I just love it – it's still long enough for me to pull back when I want to, and...." Here, Bobbie laughed. She couldn't believe her own ears: here she was, talking about hair, of all things. But it was kind of fun. All this caught Marti by surprise. My, she thought, suddenly we're seeing another side of Bobbie.

Julie must have been thinking the same thing because she said, "It makes you look so much younger." Bobbie liked hearing that and touched her hair in appreciation. Emily and Margaret voiced their approval, too. Then, before anyone could say anything else, Bobbie waved her hands as if to bat their comments away. Marti could see that it was difficult for Bobbie to receive praise. But, with time, it would get easier. Bobbie went on to explain what had happened. "You all know how boring I think charity functions are," she said. "Well, my sister's party turned out better than I could have ever imagined. The food was great, and the house looked beautiful. But I think what made the difference this time was that I decided to have a good time." She laughed once again, remembering the party and how much attention she'd received.

Almost self-consciously, she said, "For the first time in my adult life, people noticed me. I have to confess that it was a little confusing at first – I'm not used to getting so much attention." Then, feeling compelled to explain, she said, "I've always thought you had to be thin for these people to want to associate with you, but at this party I couldn't believe how many people went out of their way to be nice to me. The men even came up to talk to me. And a number of them complimented me. Some of my mother's friends even said that I looked so different, and several had the nerve to ask if I'd lost weight. Even though I've lost five or six pounds, I wouldn't have thought that was enough to make a difference in the way I look."

"Maybe," Margaret suggested, "they were trying to figure out what it was that made you look so different."

"You're probably right," Bobbie admitted. "But, it's just like them not to see beyond my weight. Still," and she couldn't repress a grin, "the best part of the whole evening was that I was in the middle of a wonderful conversation with three very attractive men when out of the corner of my eye I saw someone signaling to me. It was Garth. He'd just gotten back from his trip, read my note about meeting me at the party, and there he was. More than anything, I wanted to run right over to him – but something told me not to. So I said to myself, 'Nope, it's important that I finish this conversation.' And then before I knew it, there he was at my side. Can you believe it?" she asked. "And he interrupted to say that I looked terrific." Entranced not only with Bobbie's story, but with her animated telling of it, everyone was hanging on to her every word. "Well," Bobbie confided, "Garth simply could not take his eyes off me. I guess he liked my hair because he touched it and whispered that it was so soft. Anyway, it was like he'd never seen me before. After I introduced him to the others, we started over to my family's table and Garth said, 'Bobbie, I've never seen you this way before.' I don't know what came over me, but I said, 'Get used to it – you're looking at the new me!' And then I kept walking."

"Oh," breathed Julie, "What a perfect thing to say!"

"What happened next?" asked Emily.

"Well, we reached the family and everyone got up from the table to shake Garth's hand, and he said to them, 'Doesn't Bobbie look beautiful, tonight?' Can you imagine that?" Bobbie asked. "It's the first time anyone ever called me beautiful. My mother said, 'Is that the dress I sent you?' That's when my sister stepped in," Bobbie said, surprise showing in her voice. "Melanie said, 'I think Bobbie chose the perfect dress for her. Don't you?' Well," said Bobbie, "this was the first time my sister ever took my side. I guess that upset my mother because I could feel the tension coming from her. So, I changed the subject and she let it go. We all ended up having a really nice dinner. But, you know what? It suddenly came to me that I'd been having such a good time that I hadn't been thinking about food the way I usually do. Ordinarily, I would have been obsessed with thoughts of food from the minute I started getting ready. And that would only get worse after I got to the party. But, this time I didn't do any of that," Bobbie added. "I was eating everything that I wanted to eat, and drinking exactly what I wanted to drink. On top of that, I wasn't uncomfortably stuffed when I finished. In fact, I felt great." Again, Bobbie smiled. Never had any of them seen her so happy. Seeing their faces reflecting her own joy, Bobbie thought that even the Group was responding to her differently. So she felt comfortable in going on.

"So, this party really showed me the changes that I've made in myself over the last 18 weeks," Bobbie said. "Always before, I went to the parties only because I had to. And because I knew they were going to be boring, the only thing I had to look forward to was the food. But, now, I'm thinking that maybe I didn't have fun because my own attitude got in the way." Hearing this, Julie thought of the times she'd kept herself apart from the fun going on around her. Bobbie wasn't the only one, she thought as Bobbie wound things up with, "But this time, I really wanted to have a good time. And I did!"

Noticing how much the Group had enjoyed Bobbie's triumph with her, Marti said, "Bobbie I see you are thinking about what YOU want out of situations and doing something about it: you have taken back the power." Bobbie nodded. "You know," she said to Marti, "the first time you said that we each had the power to change things, I didn't know what you were talking about. Now, I know what that means, and how it feels, too. I made a conscious decision to have a good time at the party. So my attitude has a lot to do with what happens to me." Marti agreed.

"Maybe," she said, "this all started when you rejected the dress your mother sent over. To do all that, you had to have visualized how you wanted to look. That made everything fall into place. No wonder people noticed a change in you because it was more than your weight or your hair, or your dress. People were different with you because you were treating yourself with more value and importance. Having made the choice to have a good time, you didn't have to eat to escape boredom."

Again, Julie saw the similarity between her own attitude and Bobbie's. She'd dealt so long with the fear of the past that she hadn't been able to anticipate anything in the present and future with pleasure. Margaret, reviewing her own week, saw the wisdom in Marti's words, too. And Bobbie was in enthusiastic agreement. "It feels so good to be on the right track. While I haven't lost as much weight as I wanted and I know that I'm not finished with what needs to be done, I'm definitely going on to Phase Two." Rewarded with a quick smile from Julie, Bobbie smiled back. Kate wished that she could be that sure about herself. With nothing good to report when it was her turn, she wished she could get up and leave right now. But there was no way that she could. Besides, she was off the hook for a few more minutes because Julie volunteered to be next.

"One of the changes I've seen in myself is that I'm not thinking about food all the time. So, my food has changed a great deal; I don't eat the kids' leftovers, I don't raid the refrigerator, and I can't remember the last time I ate ding-dongs. How did I ever eat that stuff? It upsets my stomach now." Turning to Marti, she said, "You know, now that I think about it, I'm not using food to make myself feel better. Not even when I got a card in the mail from my mother this week." Recalling this, Julie explained, "Always before, I couldn't bear to open anything from her without putting something in my mouth. But, this time, food didn't even cross my mind – even when Mom really stuck it to me. The card was a belated birthday greeting – one of those mushy daughter cards. The only thing she wrote was that she missed me something terrible. She signed it, 'Love you, Mother; let's get together soon.'" Throwing up her hands, Julie said to the Group, "It's like, suddenly, we don't have a problem. She has no idea what's going on!"

"Well," Emily remarked, "your mother is only doing what she's done most of your life."

"I know," said Julie. "She is trying to manipulate me back into playing her game. And she's using all of her old tricks to get me to do what she wants. Only, I refuse to do it because I'll end up feeling hurt and angry. But I know that Mom is going to have a hard time with this because she's always found a way to get me involved again. Not this time – I'm realizing that she has to be responsible for her life." Listening to herself, Julie knew that she sounded a lot tougher than she really was. Would she ever get over feeling guilty?

Emily spoke up. "Good for you, Julie: it's a no-win situation because you always end up feeling terrible when you can't make your mother's problems go away."

"Problems that were never yours to begin with," added Margaret.

Julie replied with a broad smile; how wonderful it was to have people around who really understood. "I think it's time that I write another letter to my mother – and this time mail it," she said. "I want to thank all of you. You've all really helped me to keep my new boundaries with my mother, and that's something I've never been able to do before." Turning her attention to her notebook, Julie reported, "I wrote down some of the other changes I've seen in myself: one is that my food is really changing and I've lost weight. But I still don't know why I eat when I'm not physically hungry. I know that there are more things that I need to do. So I'm going on to Phase Two." Then Marti, who remembered all too well the old, fearful, silent Julie, said, "I have seen many changes in you, Julie. But the biggest one is your willingness to share your thoughts and feelings with the rest of us. I know that was very difficult for you to do." Margaret couldn't help agreeing. "You used to be so quiet and shy, and now you speak right up. You really have a lot to say!"

"I'm even surprising myself," answered Julie. "It's been an eye-opening 18 weeks!" Then, smiling around at all of them, Julie said, "That's all there is to tell, for now."

"I guess I'll go next," Emily offered. "This week brought up a number of mixed emotions for me. I talked with my parents, letting them know what my boundaries are in my house and with my food." Although no one said anything, Bobbie's blink illustrated her surprise, while Julie's gasp and Margaret's silent applause showed approval. Emily did not, however, respond to this with a smile. Everyone knew why when she said, "The minute I started, my father did his usual thing by getting up and leaving the room. He said that he had to go to the bathroom, but I knew that he wouldn't be coming back. So there I was, giving my speech to my mother. I told her exactly how I felt about her interference and saw her body stiffen. That is what I'd been dreading and she didn't disappoint me. In her sternest voice, she said, 'You have always been our most ungrateful child, and I was only trying to help you.' For a minute, you could have cut the silence with a knife. Then she turned around and headed for the door. You know, it was the oddest thing – all of a sudden there was a cement wall separating us; one that allowed her to act as if I no longer existed." Margaret found it hard to believe that parents really behaved this way. "I can't believe she said that!"

"Me either," Bobbie echoed. Julie said, "What a cruel thing to say!" The others shook their heads in disbelief. But Marti drew the attention back to Emily by asking her, "What feelings came up for you when that happened?"

Immediately, Emily's eyes filled. "I felt like a child again, not being able to get my parents to listen to what I had to say. But why should it be any different now? The minute someone says anything my parents don't want to hear, they disconnect and the barriers come up. At that point, it's hopeless. But just then my son walked in. I must have looked upset because he asked if I was all right. You know, hearing his boyish voice started me thinking: I'm not a helpless little girl anymore, whether my parents want to see me that way or not." Then, seeing heads all around the table nodding in unanimity, Emily was able to muster a smile through her tears. She continued, "I heard them coming down the stairs. There they were, suitcases in hand. And my father said in his coldest voice, 'We've obviously overstayed our welcome here,' and my mother announced, 'We've been invited to stay with your brother!' At that point, I didn't know whether to laugh or cry. Then my husband came in the front door. It took him a minute to figure out what was going on, so I gave him a look that said I'd explain everything later. Right away, he walked over and put his arm around my shoulders. Without saying a thing, we watched my parents stomp out the front door. But, what's funny," Emily said, "is that I'd always feared that if my parents abandoned me, I'd curl up and die. But, amazingly, I didn't feel that way at all. And I didn't die, either." Wiping her eyes, Emily said, "Instead, I felt kind of relieved." Caught up in her own storytelling, Emily was unaware of the immense empathy the others were feeling. She went on. "When we told the kids that Grandma and Grandpa had left, my son let out a victory yell. He said that he was glad to have his room back. My daughter was a little more tactful and asked if I was okay with them leaving. When I assured her that I was, she said, 'Things can get back to normal, now.' Later, I talked with my brother, who was pretty eager to know what happened; his wife had called him at work to say that Mom and Dad were waiting for him in the spare bedroom. But, even when he got home, they weren't talking. When I explained what happened, he said, 'Don't feel bad – they've always been that way!' That made me feel better. However, after I hung up, I couldn't help feeling a little guilty: it was my fault that Mom and Dad left."

Bobbie said, "It's not your fault. Besides, it's someone else's turn to take care of your parents." Emily, feeling less remorseful now, went on. "After all that, I felt like I needed to do something physical, so I went into the kitchen and started putting everything back the way I like it. I went through all the cupboards, freezer, and refrigerator to get rid of every bit of diet food my mother had pressured me into buying. When I was finished," Emily smiled, "everything looked wonderful." Throwing her arms wide, she said, "I have my house back!"

Marti was delighted. "It took courage to confront your parents."

"And you didn't back down one bit!" Julie exclaimed. Margaret added, "I'm so proud of you!" Emily didn't know what to do with all this attention. "I guess this is a big change for me," she said, "but who knows if it did any good!"

Marti could see that Emily was about to negate any progress she had made, so she said, "Your parents aren't going to change overnight – especially since they're so set in their ways and they don't acknowledge that there's a problem. It sounds like they're having a nice little tantrum to punish you for disagreeing with them. Or, maybe they can't deal with someone else's truth. The important thing is that you have started the process of changing your relationship with them by saying what you want them to know." Waiting for Emily's nod, indicating that she understood, Marti continued with, "Having made the changes to establish an adult to adult relationship with your parents, it's now up to them to either join you in the process, or not. Either way, you will be able to deal with it." Not so sure, Emily thought, I hope so. Aloud, she admitted, "No one in my family has ever stood up to my parents before, so it kind of worries me about what's going to happen next."

Marti asked a question. "Did you notice any difference in your food after they left?" Emily replied, "As a matter of fact, I have to admit that I had some misgivings about getting rid of all that diet stuff. After doing it, I realized that in throwing it out, I was saying that I wasn't going to eat it ever, ever again."

Marti asked, "What did that feel like?"

"It felt good!" Emily said. "And it still feels good!"

"Emily, when we first started, you admitted that you lived a double life. On the outside, everyone saw you eating diet food. But, when nobody was looking, you ate the foods you really wanted. Now, it's as if you're saying, I don't care what anyone thinks, I'm going to eat what my body wants to eat – I'm taking back the power to make my own choices!"

Validated, Emily said, "Well, this past week, I've learned that when there's diet food around, I go unconscious and then I feel deprived, and then I start eating and can't stop. With the diet food gone, I don't feel deprived. I feel like I can eat whatever my body wants. So I'm eating differently because the focus is on what my body is hungry for. And that's what I'm trying to satisfy." Marti observed, "Sounds like no one can tell you what to eat anymore."

211

"I just hope I can keep it up!" Emily said. "Last week when I realized I hadn't lost any weight, I wasn't sure that I should go on to Phase Two. Now, I know that I have to continue. Losing the weight isn't the most important thing to me anymore. That's always been my mother's objective. What's important to me is that I learn to give myself the things that I need and want without shame, or guilt."

"That's a wonderful goal," Marti confirmed.

"Well," Emily said, "the biggest thing I've learned is that thin isn't everything! I know now that my weight is here for a reason, and I'm going to have to keep working through that before I can let it go. Realizing that it's important that I have a good time along with everyone else helps me to entertain without becoming totally exhausted," she added. "I'm excited about all the changes in my life, even the discovery that I hate my job. Now, I'm thrilled to be considering going back to school. That's made me feel closer to my husband because he supports whatever I want to do." Nodding her understanding, Marti said, "Thank you, Emily. Now, who would like to go next?"

Margaret raised her hand and announced, "I will. I finally had a talk with my son, and it didn't turned out the way I thought it would." In the moment between that statement and Margaret's continuing, Bobbie had to ask herself if anything ever did. Margaret continued, explaining, "I took what I'd written down last week and practiced until I knew it forward and back. Unfortunately, my son's responses weren't what I expected. That wasn't necessarily bad," she hurried on to assure them.

"It just caught me by surprise. When I was finished, he looked at me with this blank stare. The silence felt like hours, but it was probably only a few minutes. When he finally found his voice, he said that he'd never realized how much I expected of him. Then he asked if I wanted him to leave. When I reassured him that he was still welcome, he grinned at me and said that he had to meet some people – like the conversation was over. So I said that when he got back, we'd finish the conversation. I ended up feeling frustrated because nothing got resolved. Then I felt guilty – how could he ever think that I'd throw him out? But there wasn't much I could do about it except wait.

When he got back, we sat down to talk. By then he had plenty to say, mostly about not being able to guarantee that he'd have a job by graduation. That seemed to be all that he remembered from our first conversation. So I pulled out my list and showed it to him. He couldn't believe that I'd actually written it down. He said, 'I've been here for two years. If all this has been bothering you, why didn't you say something earlier?' I realized that I should have said something earlier, but it wasn't until I started taking this class that I could see what was happening. It's come to me that one of the reasons he's been so immature is that I've been treating him like a child. So that's what I said. I told him that this affected everyone, including his relationship with his daughter. Then," Margaret said, "Donnie asked a question I never anticipated, 'What does Dad think about all of this?' he asked. "As if what I wanted didn't matter! Donnie probably said it to shut me up, but it didn't work because I said, 'Let's ask him.' What he didn't know is that I'd already explained my concerns to Bob. I always tried to keep Bob informed about any problems I had with the kids, but he was always too busy to get involved. So when he came into the kitchen, I could tell that he was a little uncomfortable. And my son was suddenly very nervous.

"Bob started right in with, 'It's time for you to grow up! You're a father now, and you have a child who depends on you.' When Donnie said that he wasn't sure that he could get a job that quickly, Bob said that he'd get him a list of connections he could make. It was a very touching moment. When you have a father whose never been around for baseball games and all that stuff, you don't expect him to be there when you really need him. There Bob was, helping him with a problem. On top of that, Bob said, 'Don, if you don't have a job lined up by graduation, we'll get together again and talk about it.' I was pleased that Bob would come up with a solution," Margaret said, "and surprised when he called Donnie 'Don.' That's when it occurred to me that Donnie is a boy's name. So, now, I'm calling him Don, too. Don promised to spend more time with his daughter and take better care of his things. So far," she added, "he's doing a pretty good job. I don't know how long it'll last, but if he slacks off, I'll just have to talk to him again." Then a smile spread over her face. "I can have his father talk to him, too."

"You did a great job," Marti said, "of getting everyone to talk about this problem. It sounds like you really were able to make them understand what you expect. In the process, everyone in your family grew. Including Bob in on the problem and its solution makes him a more active part of the family. For Don, it had to be a shock to hear you address him adult-to-adult, but it gives him the feeling that you have respect for, and confidence in, him. When parents assume that their children can do something, they usually can!"

"I hope you're right," said Margaret. "As you said to Emily, when you change, others begin to make changes, too. But what's more important for me right now is that I finally let everyone know how I feel."

"Things are changing all around you," Marti remarked. "Is any of it affecting your food?" Margaret laughed. "I'll say!" she said. "Bob has been working at home for the last few days. Every afternoon I buzz him to ask when he thinks he's going to be hungry for dinner. He always says the same thing – 'Whenever you want!' Whenever I want?" she asked. "All these years I thought he expected dinner at the same time. Now, it appears that he doesn't really care." Hearing the mystification in Margaret's voice, Marti couldn't help but think that it was amazing how much people discovered when they started communicating with one another. For Margaret that certainly was true, because she was saying, "Then when I asked him what he wanted to eat, I got the same answer – it didn't really matter. So I started fixing things that I wanted to eat. You know what? Most of the time he's pretty happy with whatever I fix – although he still needs his meat and potatoes every night. I'm discovering that my body wants more vegetables and fruits, so I've been trying new recipes. Who would have thought!"

Turning to the Group, Marti said, "What Margaret discovered is that her assumptions were inaccurate. We all need to make efforts to communicate with those closest to us because our needs and wants and desires change as we grow older."

Hearing this, Bobbie could relate because she'd been looking at things differently, too. Not that she'd started cooking – she didn't know if she'd ever want to do that. But she had started experimenting with those meals you could buy now at grocery stores. Meanwhile, Marti was continuing. "Good for you, Margaret, for trying something new." To the others, she said, "It's important to experiment with different recipes and foods because it gives us so many more choices. Frequently, we hear women say that they're bored with food. Nothing sounds good, nothing tastes good, and it no longer satisfies their bodies. What we've found out is that sometimes, boredom comes from craving something you haven't tasted yet. So, exploring unfamiliar foods and new recipes helps identify the tastes and textures your body wants." Listening, Julie thought that it might be well and good for Margaret to embrace vegetables and fruit, but it sounded like diet food to her.

"Another good change," Margaret went on, "is that I'm walking more. I don't drive the car down to the mailbox anymore," she said. "I walk down because I realize that when I do that, I feel better." Then, she added, "It's not very far!" With everyone else having taken their turn, Kate knew she could delay no longer.

Reluctantly, she said, "I don't have much to report except our lawyer convinced Ed that he should go into a rehab program, and he did. This means that he and I won't see each other for a couple of weeks – which is probably just as well because I know that he's mad at me for leaving him in jail. As uncertain as everything is, I'm finding that it's a relief not to have to deal every day with his anger, his drinking, or his spending. Of course, I don't know how we're going to pay our part of the rehab costs, but at least I won't have to guess what his credit charges are going to be this month."

Margaret, wanting to give Kate some hope, suggested, "Now that Ed is getting help and won't be drinking, maybe he'll stop drinking for good."

"Who knows," Kate said, still deflated. "But, you're right, there's hope. It's been suggested that I start going to Alanon, and I'm thinking about it."

Tying that in with food, Marti asked, "How did all of this affect your food this week?"

Kate had a ready answer. "Surprisingly, I haven't pigged out like I used to. But I honestly haven't had the urge."

Marti summarized, "It's really hard to want change and have to wait. But look at what you've accomplished – you've made it really clear to yourself that you want your marriage to be different, and you want your personal and businesses finances straightened out. Now, with Ed's attempt to stop drinking, there may be a greater chance for these things to work out." Ruefully, Kate agreed. Going on, Marti said, "In spite of everything that's happened, you haven't allowed any of this to throw you back into unconscious eating. You're doing a really great job!"

Hearing Marti acknowledge the changes she'd made, Kate knew that she should feel more hopeful. Things could change for the better. If they didn't, Kate knew that she would deal with them, somehow. But, the knowledge that she was capable didn't help much. Suddenly overwhelmed with all that there was to do – and how little she could control – she couldn't remember what else she'd wanted to report. Listing the changes she saw in herself was beyond her ability right now. To hide the disorientation she felt, Kate picked up her notebook and appeared to study what she'd written there. Glancing that way, Julie couldn't help but notice that the page was blank. Sensing that Kate didn't know what to say or do, Julie helped her along. "You know, Kate," she said, "I've seen a lot of changes in you since we first met. But the biggest, I think, is that you don't make light of serious things anymore. When you first started telling us what was going on in your life, I couldn't tell if you understood how serious they sounded. Now, you don't joke about those things anymore." Margaret had to agree. "Julie's right. You're far more willing to share your life and problems with us. And every one of us knows how hard that can be."

All of this praise was making Kate uneasy; she felt that she hadn't done nearly as much changing as they had. And she'd missed some classes, too. Having people accept and support her had never happened before. Used to being criticized, Kate was now afraid of disappointing these women – if she went on with the program, what would happen if she didn't divorce Ed? Feeling pressured to respond, she conceded, "I guess I have made some changes!"

Picking up on Kate's reluctance, Marti said, "In the past, whenever you dared to risk anything, you ended up feeling abused or abandoned. Trusting us was an enormous step." This compelled Kate to disclose how important everyone had become to her. "Group has become really important to me; it's the only place that I feel safe talking about things. But I don't know if I can afford going on to the next phase."

Startled to hear this, Emily wondered how Kate could NOT afford to go on – if ever anyone needed support at this time in her life, she did. But not wanting to pressure her, Emily limited herself to saying, "It wouldn't be the same without you, Kate." The rest agreed. Sensing that Kate hadn't made a decision yet, Marti wanted to take the pressure off her. So she said, "Given everything that's happened recently, it would be difficult for anyone to make a decision. So, take your time, Kate. We won't be starting again for two weeks. If you need to talk, just give me a call."

How understanding they all were, Kate thought, wondering what she wanted more, to hug everyone or to put her head down and howl out her frustration and fear. Thank heaven Marti had given her two weeks to think about it. With Ed gone, she had time to herself to think. Time to get more information about their finances, and time to make short- and long-range decisions. Marti interrupted her thoughts again. "The other big change that you've made is that you're allowing yourself to sit with your feelings rather than using food to stuff them down."

Still uneasy with all this positive attention, Kate did not reply. Wanting her turn to end as quickly as possible, she said, "Thank you," and glanced down at the table. Marti got the message. Understanding that Kate was finished, she announced that it was time start the final part of the meeting. Everyone adjusted their positions, wondering what was coming next.

Circling the table, Marti looked at each one, and said, "Because endings are just as important as beginnings, we mark the end of these first 18 weeks with a ceremony. Let's begin by taking out the stationery you were asked to bring." As everyone began reaching into their purses, Bobbie panicked. Stationery! How could she have forgotten? But then common sense told her not to fear. She always had at least one prescription pad with her. Searching around in her purse, she found it.

"At the top," Marti was saying, "put today's date. Below it, as if you were writing a letter, write Dear, and then write your own name." Baffled, everyone did as they were told. Then Marti continued. "Each of us is going to write on your paper one change we've seen in you since the program started. When you are finished, pass the paper on to the person on your right. When you get your own paper back, please hand it to me." For the next 15 minutes, nothing was said. In the silence, there was only the scratch of pens and pencils. When everyone was finished, Marti took their pages and left the room. No one knew what to make of this. A few minutes later, the therapist was back with five beautiful red roses. "Everyone please stand," Marti said. When they had, she moved to Bobbie's side, saying, "I'd like to present these to you, Bobbie, as an acknowledgment of your hard work and accomplishments." Handing Bobbie a rose and returning her paper, Marti was touched when the Group broke into spontaneous applause. Pausing long enough for the physician to enjoy this acknowledgment, Marti then moved on to say the same thing to Emily, and the group applauded again. As they did for Margaret, Kate, and Julie. Standing there, each felt a sense of pride that they'd stuck it out for so long. Hearing the changes others had witnessed, and now receiving written confirmation of those changes, filled them with emotion. When Bobbie and Kate saw the others hug one another, they felt a little uneasy about doing it, too. Awkward until Emily, Margaret, and Julie turned to them, Bobbie thought what the heck and hugged back. Kate was so standoffish, but Julie really wanted to hug her. So taking the risk, she held out her arms and put her arms around Kate. Giving Julie a quick hug in return, Kate made a dash for the door. The last thing she wanted was for someone to see her vulnerability.

On the way out the door, Margaret was thinking how lovely an ending this was. While each of them had been too shy to read what the others had written right then, they had very carefully put the papers away to read later when they were alone. Out in the parking lot, Kate did not look back for a very good reason. By now, her entire face was smeared with tears. What was she going to do, she cried, about anything?

Dear Kate,

It took a lot of courage to admit that you were not happy in your marriage. You deserve to have what you want.   Bobbie

I CAN'T TELL YOU HOW I ADMIRE THE WAY YOU HAVE KEPT IT TOGETHER IN SPITE OF EVERYTHING THAT'S HAPPENED. I HOPE YOU WON'T GIVE UP. I VALUE YOUR COMMENTS IN GROUP.   JULIE

It's really great to see how you are not letting your feelings about Ed make you binge late at night anymore. You are a very important part of our group and I hope to see you when group meets again.   Emily

I'm proud of you for remembering that you mattered at a time that it would have been so easy to isolate. You've come a long way in making the connections between feeling worthless and compulsive eating and shopping. Keep up the good work and remember that you are always worth being first on your list of things to take care of.   Marti

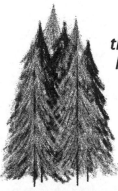

Even though you have been going through a hard time with Ed, you have not lost sight of yourself. I know that if you keep working on it, the answers will come and it will all turn out for the best in the end.

Margaret

DEAR JULIE,

It's exciting to see the changes you have made in how you think about food. You are really eating differently especially around your mother. Emily

While the changes you have made in your food have been mostly internal, the effects have been dramatic. By putting food in a different place, you have been able to make your relationships more satisfying. You took the chance to share what really happens with your mother and brother. You have gotten the support to make changes in those relationships and have been able to let go of the shame and responsibility of their lives.
Marti

I know it was hard for you to open up and trust us. But you did and I want you to know that your input has been really important to me. Margaret

I really admire how you worked through your finances with your husband. I know it was hard because you had to face your worst fear - divorce!
Kate

You should be proud of yourself for establishing and sticking to your limits with your kids and your mother! Bobbie

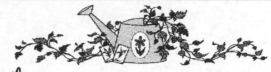

Dear Emily,

In making connections between feeling deprived and bingeing, you have started to identify the other hungers in your life professionally and personally. You are making a lot of changes and it's hard to see right now how this all relates to being at your natural body weight. You have been so aware of what you want and need in order to not feel deprived, I have confidence that the choices you are making will ultimately lead you to where you want to be.   Marti

No one can tell you what to eat anymore! Your days of living a double life are over.
                                    Margaret

I'm really proud of you for confronting your parents and it's good to see that you feel that you deserve more than your diet food!   Kate

You took a big risk changing how you deal with your mother. I know you love to entertain but it's good to hear that you want to have a good time too.
                                    Bobbie

I THINK IT'S REALLY WONDERFUL THAT YOU DECIDED TO CHANGE YOUR CAREER AND GO BACK TO SCHOOL TO BE A LAWYER. HOW EXCITING!   JULIE

<u>Bobbie Boone, M.D.</u>
County Hospital

DATE _____

NAME_____ DOB_____

ADDRESS_____

℞ : **Dear Bobbie,**

WISH I COULD HAVE SEEN GARTH'S FACE WHEN HE SAW THE NEW YOU! COLOR, STYLE AND ATTITUDE – YOU REALLY FOUND A WAY TO MAKE IT FUN FOR YOU!

JULIE

It was so good to see you take the time to do what is important to you. I've really come to appreciate your presence in the group.

Emily

It has been such a pleasure to watch you gain insight and compassion for yourself. The group has really benefited from you sharing your feelings and process. You've really made incredible progress in terms of taking time for you. You discovered the power of your thoughts on things and how it changes the way you experience your food. *Marti*

It was a big risk to talk to Garth about what you really want from him. Talking to him is the only way you will be able to know if the relationship is going to work for you.   Margaret

P.S. I really love your haircut!

I can't believe the transformation you have made. It's good to see the real Bobbie come out.

Kate

DOCTOR_____ REFILLS 1 2 3 4 5 6 PRN

M

Dear Margaret,

I admire your courage in making the connection between what happened to you as a child and your food. You are a special lady! Kate

I have a lot of respect for the way you have started to handle your relationship with your son and your husband.　　Bobbie

I REALLY ADMIRE THE WAY YOU HAVE CHANGED YOUR HOUSE TO MAKE IT FEEL LIKE SOME PLACE SPECIAL FOR YOU. I KNOW IT WAS HARD TO TELL YOUR HUSBAND WHAT YOU WANTED.　　JULIE

When you made the connection between loneliness and your eating, it was not only powerful for you but powerful to me as well. It's so nice to see you value what you want in the things you do these days.　　Emily

I'm so proud of you for staying with your feelings and not rushing to fill the emptiness inaccurately. You're doing a good job of letting your feelings and desires be known. I'm confident that with the changes you are making with your food and everything else that when you are ready, it will be safe to let the weight come off.　　Marti

Dear Reader,

As you may have guessed we are not finished with Bobbie, Kate, Julie, Margaret, and Emily. Follow their lives as they continue their journey to permanent weight loss in future books.

We congratulate you for taking the first step in making the emotional connection to your weight. This is just the first of many steps in your journey. Remember, you are the expert of your body and the answers are there within each one of you.

We want you to know that we are here to help you in any way we can to support your process of discovering the connection between feelings, food, and weight loss. In addition to this book, DIETLESS™ *has other services that are available to you:*

The **DIETLESS** Newsletter

The **DIETLESS** Conference

DIETLESS Groups in your area

If you would like more information about these services, please feel free to contact us:

Telephone: 800-643-7711 • Fax: 619-463-8986

E-mail: dietless@dietless.com • Web page : www.dietless.com

We wish you all the best,

You deserve no less!!

Carol & Joanna